AF598219

50545314 No:7400023391 Cl:821.59
WITHDRAWN
GARTH S/DISPENSARY
Ed: 00 Date: 1975 Vol: 000 Loc: 00 Lo: 0

GC

A f

T

The Dispensary

By Samuel Garth

with

A Short Account of the Proceedings of the College of Physicians, London, in Relation to the Sick Poor (1697)

and

Claremont (1715)

Facsimile Reproductions with an Introduction By Jo Allen Bradham

Scholars' Facsimiles & Reprints
Delmar, New York 1975

Published by Scholars' Facsimiles & Reprints, Inc.,
Delmar, New York 12054

Printed in the United States of America

Reproduced from copies in The British Library, London, and the National Library of Medicine, Bethesda, Maryland

Library of Congress Cataloging in Publication Data

Garth, Sir Samuel, 1661–1719.
The dispensary (1725) with A short account of the proceedings of the College of Physicians, London, in relation to the sick poor (1697) and Claremont (1715).

Photoreprint ed.
Includes bibliographical references.
1. Royal College of Physicians of London. I. Title: The dispensary.
PR3471.G3A6 1975 821'.5 74-23391
ISBN 0-8201-1145-7

Introduction

Dr. Johnson, in *Lives of the Poets,* pronounces Sir Samuel Garth's *Dispensary* lacking in "poetical ardour"; George Sherburn describes it as "now unreadeable";[1] and R. P. Bond dismisses it as "doubly dull."[2] Even John Dennis, who was a close friend of Garth's and who generally reached critical appraisals quite opposite to the consensus, found *The Dispensary* only a "beautiful libel."[3] On the other hand, Alexander Pope praised it, not only by saying that each alteration was an improvement,[4] but also by lifting thinly disguised lines for use in his own poetry. Pope's reasons for adulation were gratitude, friendship, and repayment of compliments, not objective analysis, for Garth had encouraged, advised, and helped establish the young Pope. Apparently no one—save Pope—has ever applauded *The Dispensary;* nevertheless, no student of Augustan letters can disregard it.

Perhaps *The Dispensary* is best viewed as a repository of the technique, if not the genius, of the age that produced it, as a vital footnote documenting the methods that writers other than Garth turned into art. One values Garth's poem not for its whole but for its parts—the conventions of the mock-heroic, the architectonics of the closed couplet, and the public nature of Augustan poetry. The sum of its parts is, in this case, greater than the whole.

Like the more famous Restoration and eighteenth-century mock-heroics, *The Dispensary* had its inception in a public dispute and drew its cast from public men with whom the author was personally involved. In 1688 the London College of Physicians first directed free apothecary service as well as medical care for the indigent; by 1696 financial support was obtained and service extended. For various reasons (primarily the opposition of the apothecaries), the project was short-lived, and only Garth's poem remains to explore the attitudes and conflicts of the men concerned with the medical program. That the poem is public in nature and appeared in response to particular contemporary events is stressed by Garth himself in his Preface. There he refers to *A Short Account of the Proceedings of the College of Physicians, London, in Relation to the Sick Poor,* a "treatise"—as he styles it—which traces the motives of the College of Physicians, describes the resolutions adopted by that body, and prints both the formal response by the Society of Apothecaries and the ensuing rejoinder from the College.

The *Short Account,* as Garth indicates, gives the facts of the adventure in charity, but the tone and diction occasionally indicate that spite and jealousy rather than professional charity defined the relationship between the doctor and the dispenser. The indictment of the apothecaries within the mock-heroic has its roots in the narrative account in which the physicians claim their rivals offer "proof of their great Ambition to meddle with what belongs not to them, to set themselves up for Physicians, and run themselves into practice upon pretence of Charity to the Poor . . ." (p. 13). Although only an expository pamphlet, the *Account* merges into *The Dispensary.* The two works (both reprinted in this edition) offer a striking case study of satire's emergence from and response to society's causes.

The *Account* not only documents the social and professional milieu of *The Dispensary* but also explains the topical and highly limited nature of Garth's artistic interpretation. Though initially much in demand, the poem slipped from popular and critical attention early in the second half of the eighteenth century. The years between 1699 and 1768 saw eleven authorized editions, at least one which was unauthorized, and various reprintings. So great was the popular demand that the first three editions appeared in the same year (1699). The second, a much expanded version of the first, introduced the prefatory explanation, the dedication to Anthony Henley, Garth's fellow Kit-Kat and encourager of satire, and the four complimentary letters to the doctor-poet.

The creation and evolution of the *Compleat Key to The Dispensary* further indicate the early popularity of Garth's exposé of a medical scandal. First issued to explain the sixth edition, the *Key* changed as the text changed, glossing the different versions as they appeared.

After the eleventh edition of 1768, there were no others until Wilhelm Josef Leicht, using the 1714 seventh edition as his source, prepared one in 1905 with German notes and commentary as part of the *Englische Textbibliothek* series. Footnotes in Leicht's volume give variant readings for all editions.

These facts of publication not only establish the original popularity of the poem, but also show that Garth's *magnum opus* has been buried for the English audience for roughly two hundred years, that is, since the 1768 printing. There has been another type of burial for the work, however. Editions of Pope at the most emphasize and at the least allude to *The Dispensary* in footnotes; and studies of other authors and of the age intimate the debt to Samuel Garth. *The Dispensary* has been both known, thanks to the apparatus of scholarly notation, and unknown because of its out-of-print status and highly topical subject. One must know it in full, not in footnote fashion, if his evaluation of Pope is to be accurate; his understanding of the mock-heroic, to be thoroughgoing; and his knowledge of couplet prosody, to be complete. The technique of Garth's poem may not be easily dismissed, even though a seventeenth-century quarrel between physicians and apothecaries is now nothing.

A physician, Garth brought to poetry neither originality nor the conviction that the Muses guided him. He was a man of letters and learning, but he made no effort to pass as an artist divinely inspired. One of his literary projects was a new translation and edition of Ovid's *Metamorphoses*. Garth selected the persons to translate the various books, rendered Book Fourteen himself, and issued a Preface which outlines his literary values. This Preface projects a mind that is highly competent, knowledgeable, and thorough but neither original nor daring. He will, he promises, "take notice of some of the beauties . . . and also of the faults, and particular affectations." [5] That Garth, having initiated the project and selected translators, still promises that he "shall not pretend to impose [his] opinions on others" (xxv), indicates a temperament from which one would hardly expect a literary revolution.

There is, nevertheless, merit in Garth's criticism; and the Preface to Ovid remains valuable because it provides a standard of literary knowledge against which to measure *The Dispensary* and the verse epistle *Claremont*. Speaking of Ovid, Garth claims that art is to be praised primarily for "redundance of wit, justness of comparison, elegance of description" (xxv). These are the traits salient—if not consistently maintained—in *The Dispensary*. Thus, one may conclude that what Garth admired in art, he was capable of effecting in art. One persuasive example of wit, fine comparison, and effective description, as appropriate to grim disease and the satiric mode, comes in Canto VI. Here, fever and corruption, personified and functioning as characters, move and threaten. Their presentation, in terms of setting, image, and emotional impact, recalls the old parade of sins. Such a linking adds to the natural horror, as these ghastly figures evoke death, both symbolically and literally.

Garth expected literature to evidence propriety of language and metaphor and to have what he termed an "instructive excellence of the morals" (xxix). This emphasis explains both the strength and the failure of *The Dispensary,* the many occasions where artistic integrity is sacrificed to make the point of charity, civic duty of physicians, and the high calling and creed of a doctor. The Preface to *The Dispensary,* in acknowledging the faults of the poem, makes it clear that the philanthropic medical cause was more important in Garth's intention and construction than was poetic excellence.

Even the fact that *The Dispensary* has never prompted diverse interpretation may be understood in terms of Garth's artistic principles, exactly the principles that one might expect from a man trained in the sciences. He favored obvious art, clear and unequivocal. Writing about Ovid, Garth argues: "Allegories should be obvious, and not like meteors in the air, which represent a different figure to every different eye. Now they are armies of soldiers; now flocks of sheep; and by and by nothing" (xiviii). The directness of *The Dispensary* in both its technique and its meaning grows from Garth's stated theory of composition. The doctor-poet's critical, artistic, and professional position was one of conservatism; neither "timorousness" nor "wanton abandon," two terms from his criticism, is acceptable.

Garth's mock-epic evidences sound method and considerable verve yet misses brilliance. This imbalance is consistent with other aspects of Garth's career. As a physician, he was of solid reputation, good counsel, and very much in demand; Lady Mary, Gay, and Steele make specific reference to his medical skill. Nevertheless, he made no contributions to medical science, even though his lecture on the respiratory process was praised in his own time. He used what was well known, but the profession was not changed by his presence. As artist, Garth practiced poetry with adequacy and contemporary success, offering situations and couplets on which men like Pope could build, but creating no monument for himself.

It is proper, however, to judge Garth's poem in terms of the mock-heroics which preceded, not in terms of the more successful ones which followed and in some details built on his plan. Before 1699 there was little to illustrate the mock-heroic in England. In comparison with John Heywood's *The Spider and the Flie* (1556) with its involved religious allegory, the directness and clarity of *The Dispensary* mark a distinct improvement. Unlike the fourteenth-century *Turnament of Totenham,* attributed to Gilbery Pilkington, Garth's poem deals with the substance of life—the health of the commonweal—not the mere style of court and chivalry. *The Dispensary* helps define the mock-heroic as a social voice and social tool capable of addressing itself to major public matters. The serious theme separates *The Dispensary* from Michael

Drayton's 1627 effort in mock-heroics, *The Nimphidia,* which is a charming consideration of trivia. Longer and more ambitious than *MacFlecknoe* (1682), with which it has much in common, *The Dispensary* depends on multiple epic events, not a single dramatic episode. The epic conventions—invocation, battle, descent into the underworld, supernatural intervention, allusion, long and lofty speeches, presence of monster and near-monster, and symbolic names—find effective, if not exciting, application. Similarly, the poetic devices of balance, inversion, chiasmus, magnification coupled with diminution (both within the single line and within the verse paragraph), climactic triplet for satiric reduction, and mock-epic similies link Garth with the kind of mock-heroic Dryden wrote.

Garth acknowledged a debt to Boileau's *Lutrin,* not to an English inheritance; nevertheless the doctor-poet contributed to the English line. He tightened the structure of the mock-heroic, applied almost all the epic conventions and events in appropriate and useful ways, and made language of all dictional levels and sources an acceptable part of the mock-heroic manner. While his craftsmanship did not actually remold the genre, it honed it, freeing the form from irrelevancies of allegory, affectations of style, and trivial subject matter.

Both Garth's own statement in the Preface and the commendatory letters to the author testify that Garth's theory of satire was the conventional one of his time. His purpose is moral reformation; misinterpretation of the characters by the guilty is the fault of the reader, not the attack of the satirist:

> If the *Satyr* may appear directed at any particular Person, 'tis at such only as are presum'd to be engag'd in Dishonourable Confederacies for mean and mercenary Ends, against the Dignity of their own Profession. But it there be no such, then these Characters are but imaginary, and by consequence ought to give no Body Offence.

The present text, a reprint of the ninth edition (Dublin, 1725) has been selected because of the fullness of the *Compleat Key to the Dispensary* and because the *Key* in that edition was printed with the poem, not separately. The text of the poem is identical, except in matters of punctuation, with that of 1714, the seventh edition, the last to appear in Garth's lifetime. The *Compleat Key,* however, carries as a separate section the passages omitted from various earlier editions. For example, the first couplet omitted in preceding editions—"Why Atticus polite, Brutus severe, / Why Me——n muddy, M——que why clear" (I. 54–55)—is printed in the *Key,* not in the body of the poem. The couplet was cancelled after the sixth edition (1706), and only by using the *Key* does one have the resources to study the textual evolution of *The Dispensary*.

Seven illustrations of the action described in the poem first appeared in the 1714 edition. One engraving was at frontispiece, and another marked the title page of each canto. These engravings were not included in the 1725 Dublin edition although they were used in the 1726 London printing. Both the 1725 Dublin and the 1726 London versions are the ninth edition. The illustrations, taken from the 1726 London issue, are reprinted in this volume, one at frontispiece and the others as a unit after the *Key*.

In addition to *The Dispensary,* Garth wrote many minor poems, most of them occasional and commendatory. Of these, the longest and most important is *Claremont,* which is reprinted in this edition. Written in 1715, *Claremont,* a verse epistle in form, celebrates the Earl of Clare (Thomas Pelham-Holles, later Duke of Newcastle-Upon-Tyne and of Newcastle-under-Lyme) and his estate Claremont. Like "Cooper's Hill," "Windsor Forest," and the *Epistle to Burlington* in some features, *Claremont* combines many strains—a satiric voice especially in the opening section; medical imagery ("Murrain" [l. 162], "circulate green blood" [l. 183], "calenture of Sultry skies" [l. 243]); classical mythology; pastoralism; and courtly compliment.

Claremont, like *The Dispensary,* is a poem of admirable parts in its reliance on and illustration of various conventions and techniques. And while neither the epistle to the Earl of Clare's estate nor the mock-heroic of the Royal College of Physicians' effort in charity may be said to "Snatch a Grace beyond the Reach of Art," both remain irreplaceable tools in assessing the epistle and the mock-heroic of the eighteenth century.

JO ALLEN BRADHAM

Agnes Scott College
Decatur, Georgia

Notes

1. George Sherburn, "The Restoration and Eighteenth Century," in *A Literary History of England,* ed. Albert C. Baugh (New York: Appleton-Century-Crofts, 1948), p. 899.

2. R. P. Bond, *English Burlesque Poetry 1700–1750* (New York: Russell and Russell, 1964), p. 156.

3. John Dennis, *Critical Works,* ed. Edward Niles Hooker (Baltimore: The Johns Hopkins Press, 1943), 2: 201.

4. Samuel Johnson, "Samuel Garth," in *Lives of the English Poets,* ed. G. B. Hill (Oxford: Clarendon, 1905), 2: 64. In footnote, Hill identifies Johnson's source as *Richardsoniana.*

5. *Ovid's Metamorphoses in Fifteen Books. Translated into English Verse under the Direction of Sir Samuel Garth . . .* (Verona, Italy: Officina Bodoni, 1958), p. xxv. This is the modern edition from the "Limited Editions Club"; all subsequent references will be from this edition and cited in the text by page number.

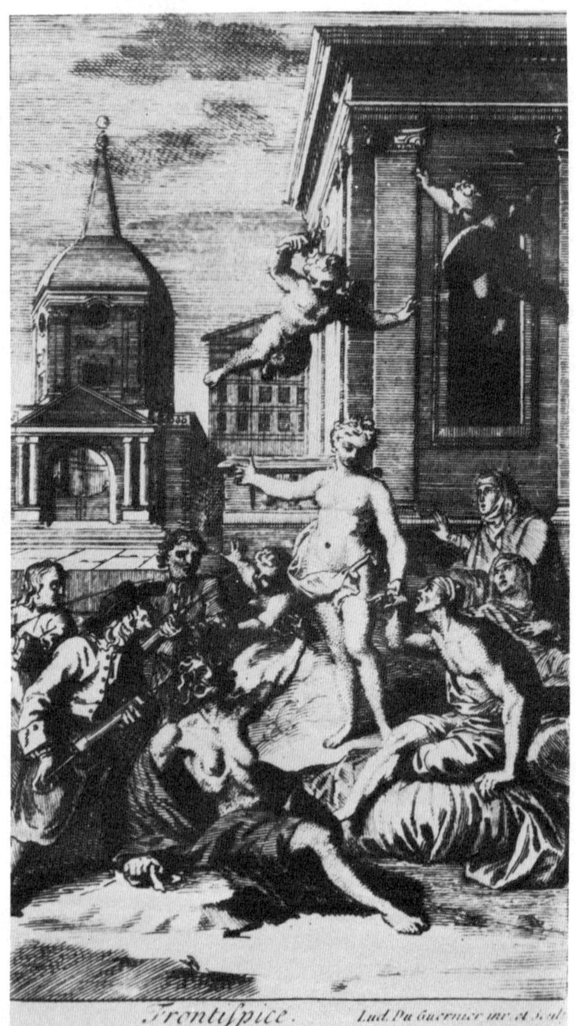

Frontispice. Lud. Du Guernier inv. et Sculp.

THE DISPENSARY. A POEM.

In Six CANTO'S.

—*Hanc veniam petimusque damusque vicissim.*
Hor. de A. P.

The Ninth Edition.

To which is added
Several Verses omitted in the late Editions, and a Compleat KEY to the whole.

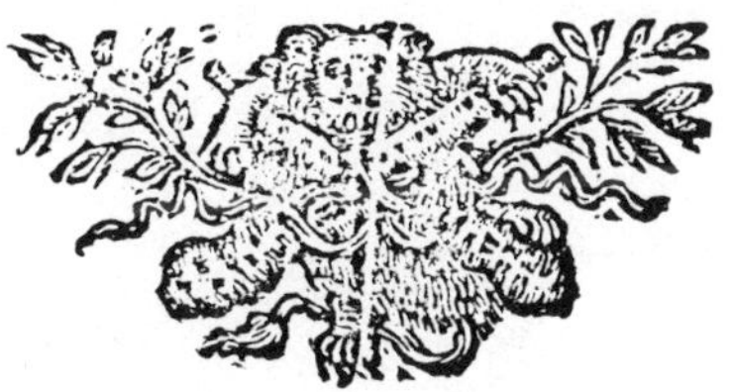

DUBLIN:
Printed by PRESSICK RIDER, and THOMAS HARBIN, for PAT. DUGAN, Bookseller, on *Cork-Hill*, MDCCXXV.

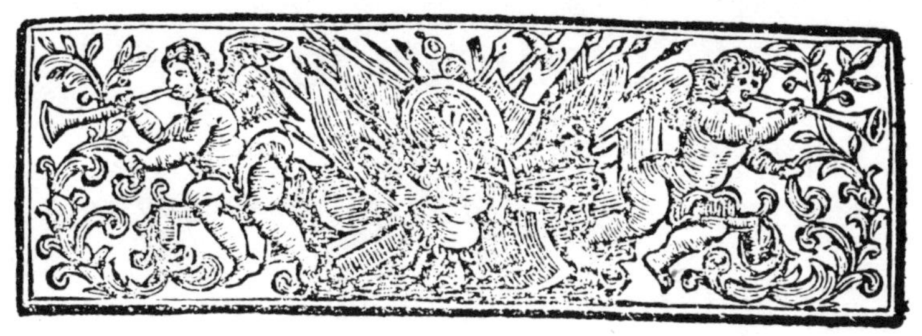

TO

Anthony Henley, *Esq;*

A MAN of Your Character can no more Prevent a Dedication, than he wou'd Encourage one; for Merit, like a Virgin's Blushes, is still most discover'd, when it labours most to be conceal'd.

'Tis hard, that to think well of You, shou'd be but Justice, and to tell You so, shou'd be an Offence: Thus rather than violate Your Modesty, I must be wanting

ing to Your other Virtues; and to gratifie One good Quality, do wrong to a Thousand.

The World generally measures our Esteem by the Ardour of our Pretences; and will scarce believe that so much Zeal in the Heart, can be consistent with so much Faintness in the Expressions; but when they reflect on your Readiness to do Good, and Your Industry to hide it; on Your Passion to oblige, and Your Pain to hear it own'd; They'll conclude, that Acknowledgments wou'd be Ungrateful to a Person, who ev'n seems to receive the Obligation he confers.

But tho' I shou'd persuade my self to be silent upon all Occasions; those more Polite Arts, which, 'till of late, have Languish'd and Decay'd, wou'd appear

appear under their present Advantages, and own You for one of their generous Restorers: Insomuch, that Sculpture now Breaths, Painting Speaks, Musick Ravishes; and as You Help to refine Our Taste, You distinguish Your Own.

Your Approbation of this Poem, is the only Exception to the Opinion the World has of Your Judgment, that ought to relish nothing so much, as what You Write Your self: But You are resolv'd to forget to be a Critick, by remembring You are a Friend. To say more, wou'd be uneasie to You; and to say less, wou'd be unjust in

Your Humble Servant.

THE

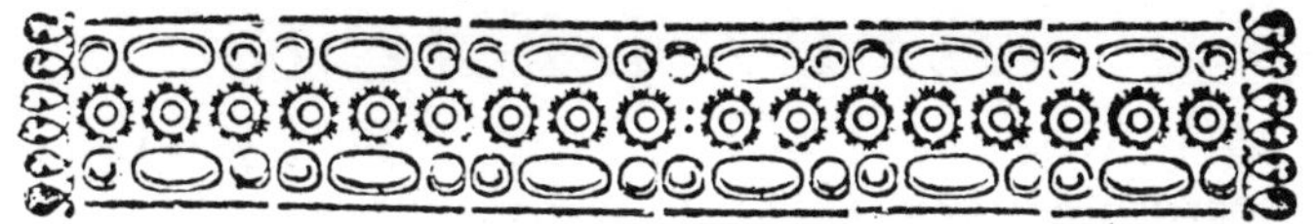

THE

PREFACE.

SINCE this following Poem in a manner ſtole into the World, I cou'd not be ſurpriz'd to find it uncorrect: Tho' I can no more ſay I was a ſtranger to its coming abroad, than I approv'd of the Publiſher's Precipitation in doing it: For a Hurry in the Execution, generally produces a Leiſure in Reflection; ſo when we run the faſteſt, we ſtumble the oftneſt. However, the Errors of the Printer have not been greater than the Candor of the Reader: And if I could but ſay the ſame of the Defects of the Author, he'd need no Juſtification againſt the Cavils of ſome furious Criticks, who, I am ſure, wou'd have been better pleas'd if they had met with more Faults.

Their Grand Objection is, That the Fury *Diſeaſe* is an improper Machine to recite Characters, and recommend the Example of preſent Writers: But tho' I had the Authority of ſome *Greek* and *Latin* Poets, upon Parallel Inſtances, to to Juſtifie the Deſign; yet, that I might not introduce any thing that ſeem'd inconſiſtent or hard, I ſtarted this Objection my ſelf, to a Gentleman very remarkable in this ſort of Criticiſm, who wou'd by no means allow that the Contrivance was forc'd, or the Conduct incongruous.

Diſeaſe is repreſented a *Fury* as well as *Envy*: She is imagin'd to be forc'd by an Incantation from her receſs; and to be reveng'd on the Exorciſt, mortifies him with an Introduction of ſeveral Perſons eminent in an Accompliſhment he has made ſome Advances in.

Nor is the Compliment leſs to any Great Genius mention'd there; ſince a very Fiend, who naturally repines at any Excellency, is forc'd to confeſs how happily They've all ſucceeded.

Their next Objection is, That I have imitated the *Lutrin* of Monſieur *Boilieau*. I muſt own I am proud of the Imputation; unleſs their Quarrel be, That I have not done it enough: But he that will give himſelf the Trouble of examining, will find I have copy'd him in nothing but in two or three Lines in the Complaint of *Moleſſe*, *Canto* II. and in one in his firſt *Canto*; the Senſe of which Line is intirely his and I could wiſh it were not the only good One in mine.

I have ſpoke to the moſt material Objections I have heard of, and ſhall tell theſe Gentlemen, that for ev'ry Fault they pretend to find in this *Poem*, I'll undertake to ſhew them two. One of theſe curious Perſons does me the Honour to ſay, He approves

approves of the Conclusion of it; but I suppose 'tis upon no other Reason but because 'tis the Conclusion. However, I shou'd not be much concern'd not to be thought Excellent in an Amusement I have very little practis'd hitherto, nor perhaps ever shall again.

Reputation of this Sort is very hard to be got, and very easie to be lost; its pursuit is painful, and its Possession is unfruitful: Nor had I ever attempted any thing in this kind, till finding the Animosities among the Members of the *College of Physicians* increasing daily (notwithstanding the frequent Exhortation of our Worthy President to the contrary) I was persuaded to attempt something of this Nature, and to endeavour to Railly some of our Disaffected Members into a Sense of their Duty, who have hitherto most obstinately oppos'd all Manner of Union; and have continu'd so unreasonably refractory, that 'was thought fit by the College, to reinforce the Observance of the Statutes by a Bond, which some of them wou'd not comply with, tho' none of 'em had refus'd the Ceremony of the Customary Oath; like some that will trust their Wives with any Body, but their Money with none. I was sorry to find there cou'd be any Constitution that was not to be cur'd without Poison, and that there shou'd be a Prospect of effecting it by a less grateful Method than Reason and Persuasion.

The Original of this Difference has been of some Standing, tho' it did not break out to Fury and Excess till the Time of Erecting the *Dispensary*, being an Apartment in the *College* set up for the Relief of the Sick Poor, and manag'd ever ſince with an Integrity and Diſintereſt ſuitable to ſo Charitable a Deſign.

If any Perſon wou'd be more fully inform'd about the Particulars of ſo Pious a Work I refer him to a Treatiſe ſet forth by the Authority of the Preſident and Cenſors, in the Year 97. 'Tis call'd *A ſhort Account of the Proceedings of the College of Phyſicians*, London, *in relation to the Sick Poor*. The Reader may there not only be inform'd of the Riſe and Progreſs of this ſo Publick an Undertaking, but alſo of the Concurrence and Encouragement it met with from the Moſt, as well as the moſt Ancient Members of the Society, notwithſtanding the vigorous Oppoſition of a few Men who thought it their Intereſt to defeat ſo laudable a Deſign.

The Intention of this Preface is not to perſuade Mankind to enter into our Quarrels, but to vindicate the Author from being cenſur'd of taking any indecent Liberty with a Faculty he has the Honour to be a Member of. If the *Satyr* may appear directed at any particular Perſon, 'tis at ſuch only as are preſum'd to be engag'd in Diſhonourable Confederacies for mean and mercenary Ends, againſt the Dignity of their own Profeſſion. But if there be no ſuch, then theſe Characters are but imaginary, and by conſequence ought to give no Body Offence.

The Deſcription of the Battel is grounded upon a Feud that happen'd in the *Diſpenſary*, betwixt a Member of the *College* with his Retinue,

and

and ſome of the Servants that attended there to diſpenſe the Medicines; and is ſo far real; tho' the Poetical Relation be fictitious. I hope no Body will think the Author too undecently reflecting thro' the whole, who being too liable to Faults himſelf, ought to be leſs ſevere upon the Miſcarriages of others. There is a Character in this trivial Performance, which the Town, I find, applies to a particular Perſon: 'Tis a Reflection which I ſhou'd be ſorry ſhou'd give Offence; being no more than what may be ſaid of any Phyſician remarkable for much Practice. The killing of numbers of Patients is ſo trite a Piece of Raillery, that it ought not to make the leaſt Impreſſion either upon the Reader, or the Perſon 'tis apply'd to; being one that I think in my Conſcience a very able Phyſician, as well as a Gentleman of extraordinary Learning. If I am hard upon any one, 'tis my Reader: But ſome Worthy Gentlemen, as remarkable for their Humanity as their Extraordinary Parts, have taken care to make him amends for it, by prefixing ſomething of their own.

I confeſs thoſe Ingenious Gentlemen have done me a great Honour; but while they deſign an imaginary Panegyrick upon me, They have made a real one upon Themſelves; and by ſaying how much this ſmall Performance exceeds ſome others, They convince the World how far it falls ſhort of Theirs.

The Copy of an Inſtrument Subſcribed by the Preſident, Cenſor, moſt of the Elects, Senior Fellows, Candidates, &c. of the College of Phyſicians, in relation to the Sick Poor.

W*Hereas the ſeveral Orders of the College of Phyſicians*, London, *for preſcribing Medicins* gratis *to the Poor Sick of the Cities of* London *and* Weſtminſter, *and Parts adjacent, as alſo the Propoſals made by the ſaid College to the Lord Mayor, Court of Aldermen and Common Council of* London, *in purſuance thereof have hitherto been ineffectual, for that no Method hath been taken to furniſh the Poor with Medicins for their Cure at low and reaſonable Rates; we therefore whoſe Names are here under-written, Fellows or Members of the ſaid College, being willing effectually to promote ſo great a Charity, by the Counſel and good Liking of the Preſident and College declared in their* Comitia, *hereby (to wit, each of us ſeverally and apart, and not the one for the other of us) do oblige our ſelves to pay to Dr.* Thomas Burwell, *Fellow and Elect of the ſaid College, the Sum of Ten Pounds a piece of Lawful Money of* England, *by ſuch Proportions, and ſuch Times as to the major Part of the Subſcribers hereto ſhall ſeem moſt convenient: Which Money when received by the ſaid Dr.* Thomas Burwell, *is to be by him expended in preparing and delivering Medicins to the Poor at their intrinſick Value, in ſuch Manner, and at ſuch Times, and by ſuch*

Orders

Orders and Directions, as by the major Part of the Subscribers hereto, shall in Writing be hereafter appointed and directed for that Purpose. In Witness whereof we have hereunto set our Hands and Seals this Twenty Second Day of December, 1696.

Tho. Millington, *Præses.*
Tho. Burwell, *Elect and Censor.*
Sam. Collins, *Elect*
Edw. Browne, *Elect*
Rich. Torless, *Elect and Censor.*
Edw. Hulse, *Elect.*
Tho. Gill, *Censor.*
Will. Dawes, *Censor.*
Jo. Hutton.
Rob. Brady.
Hans Sloane.
Richard Morton.
John Hawys.
Cha. Harel.
Rich. Robinson.
Joh. Bateman.
Walter Mills.
Dan. Coxe.
Henry Sampson.
Thomas Gibson.
Charles Goodall.
Edm. King.
Sam. Garth.
Barnh. Soame.
Denton Nicholas.
Joseph Gaylard.
John Woollaston.
Steph. Hunt.
Oliver Horseman.
Rich. Morton, *Jun.*
David Hamilton.
Hen. Morelli.
Walter Harris.
William Briggs.
Th. Colladon.
Martin Lister.
Jo. Colbatch.
Bernard Connor.
W. Cockburn.
J. le Feure.
P. Sylvestre.
Cha. Morton.
Walt. Charlton.
Phineas Fowke.
Tho. Alvery.
Rob. Gray.
John Wright.
James Drake.
Sam. Morris.
John Woodward.
. . . . Norris.
George Colebrock.
Gineod Harvey.

The Design of Printing the Subscribers Names, is to shew, that the late Undertaking has the Sanction of a College Act; and that 'tis not a Project carried on by Five or Six Members, as those that oppose it would unjustly insinuate.

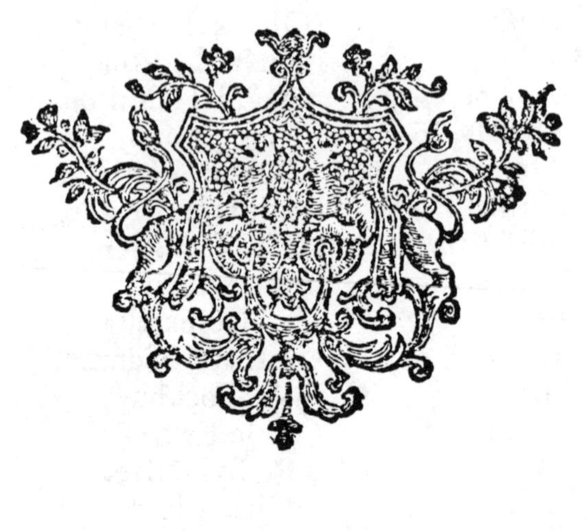

To

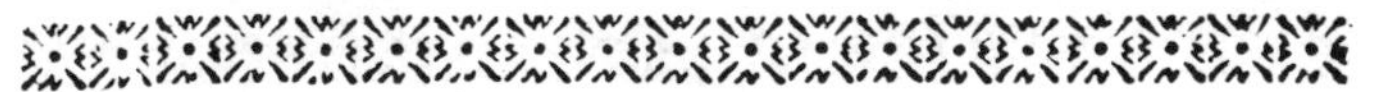

To Dr. *G—th* upon the *Dispensary.*

OH that some Genius, whose Poetick Vein,
Like *M - - - gue*'s cou'd a just Piece sustain,
Wou'd search the *Gracian* and the *Latin* Store,
And thence present thee with the purest Oar:
In lasting Numbers praise thy whole Design,
And manly Beauty of each Nervous Line:
Show how your pointed Satyr's Sterling Wit
Does only Knaves, or formal Blockheads hit;
Who're gravely Dull, *insipidly Serene*,
And carry all their Wisdom in their Mein.
Whom thus expos'd, thus strip'd of their Disguise
None will again Admire, most will Despise.
Show in what Noble Verse *Nassau* you sing,
How such a Poet's worthy such a King.
When S - - - -r's Charming Eloquence you Praise,
How loftily your Tuneful Voice you raise!
But my poor feeble Muse is as unfit
To praise, as Imitate what you have writ.
Artists alone shou'd venture to Commend
What *D - - - -s* can't Condemn, nor *D - - - -n* Mend
What must, writ with that Fire and with that Ease,
The Beaux, the Ladies and the Criticks please.

B 2 C. BOYLE.

TO MY

Friend the Author,

Desiring my

Opinion of his POEM.

ASK me not, Friend, what I Approve or blame;
Perhaps I know not why I like, or damn;
I can be pleas'd; and I dare own I am.
I read Thee over with a Lover's Eye;
Thou hast no Faults, or I no Faults can spy;
Thou art all beauty, or all blindness I.
Criticks and Aged Beaux of Fancy chaste,
Who ne'er had Fire, or else whose Fire is past,
Must Judge by Rules what they want Force to Taste.
I wou'd a Poet, like a Mistress, try,
Not by her Hair, her Hand, her Nose, her Eye;
But by some Nameless Pow'r, to give me Joy.
The Nymph has G----n's, C---l's, C---l's, Charms,
If with resistless Fires my Soul she warms,
With Balm upon her Lips, and Raptures in her Arms.
Such is thy Genius, and such Art is thine,
Some Secret Magick works in ev'ry Line;
We Judge not, but we feel the Pow'r Divine.
Where all is Just, is beauteous, and is fair,
Distinctions vanish of peculiar Air.

Lost

Lost in our Pleasure, we Enjoy in you
Lucretius, *Horace*, *S----d*, *M----gue.*
And yet 'tis thought, some Criticks in this Town,
By Rules to all, but to themselves, unknown,
Will Damn thy Verse, and Justifie their own.
Why, let them Damn: Were it not wondrous hard
Facetius *M----* and the City *B----*
So near ally'd in Learning, Wit, and Skill,
Shou'd not have leave to Judge, as well as Kill?
Nay, let them write; Let them their Forces join,
And hope the Motly Piece may Rival thine.
Safely despise their Malice, and their Toil,
Which Vulgar Ears alone will reach, and will defile.
Be it thy Gen'rous Pride to please the Best,
Whose Judgment, and whose Friendship is a Test.
With Learned *H----* thy healing Cares be join'd,
Search thoughtful *R----e* to his inmost Mind:
Unite, restore your Arts, and Save Mankind.
Whilst all the busie *M----ls* of the Town
Envy our Health, and pine away their own.
When e'er thou wou'd'st a tempting Muse engage,
Judicious *W----h* can best direct her Rage.
To *S----s*, and to *D----t* too submit,
And let their Stamp Immortalize thy Wit.
Consenting Phœbus bows, if they approve,
And Ranks thee with the foremost Bards above:
Whilst these of right the Deathless Laurel send,
Be it thy humble bus'ness to commend
The faithful, honest Man, and the well-natur'd Friend.

Chr. Codrington.

To my Friend Dr. *G—th* the Author of the *Dispensary*.

TO Praise your Healing Art would be in vain;
The Health you give, prevents the Poet's Pen.
Sufficiently confirm'd is your Renown,
And I but fill the Chorus of the Town.
That let me wave, and only now admire
The dazling Rays of your Poetick Fire.
Which its diffusive Virtue does dispense,
In flowing Verse, and elevated Sense.

The Town, which long has swallow'd foolish Verse,
Which Poetasters every where rehearse;
Will mend their Judgment now, refine their Taste,
And gather up th' Applause they throw in waste.
The Play-House shan't encourage false sublime,
Abortive Thoughts, with *Decoration-Rhime*.

The Satyr of vile Scriblers shall appear
On none, except upon themselves severe:
While yours contemns the Gall of Vulgar Spight;
And when you seem to Smile the most, you Bite.

Tho. Cheek.

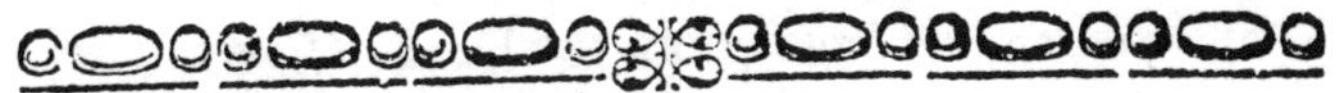

TO MY FRIEND, UPON THE DISPENSARY.

AS When the people of the Northern Zone
Find the approach of the Revolving Sun,
Pleas'd and reviv'd, They see the New born Light,
And dread no more Eternity of Night:

Thus we, who lately as of Summer's Heat
Have felt a Dearth of Poetry and Wit;
Once fear'd, *Apollo* would return no more
From warmer Climes, to an ungrateful Shore.
But You, the Fav'rite of the Tuneful Nine,
Have made the God in his full Lustre shine;
Our Night have chang'd into a glorious Day;
And reach'd Perfection in your first Essay:
So the young Eagle that his Force would try,
Faces the Sun, and tow'rs it to the Sky.

Others proceed to Art by slow Degrees,
Aukward at first, at length they faintly please.
And still whate'er their first Efforts Produce,
'Tis an abortive, or an Infant Muse.

Whilst

Whilst yours, like *Pallas* from the Head of *Jove*,
Steps out full grown, With Noblest Pace to move,
What ancient Poets to their Subjects owe,
Is here inverted, and this owes to you:
You found it little, but have made it great;
They could describe, but you alone Create.

Now let your Muse rise with expanded Wings,
To sing the Fate of Empires, and of Kings;
Great *WILLIAM*'s Victories she'll next rehearse,
And raise a Trophy of Immortal Verse:
Thus to your Art proportion the Design,
And mighty things with mighty Numbers join,
A Second *Namur*, or a future *Boyne*.

H. BLOUNT.

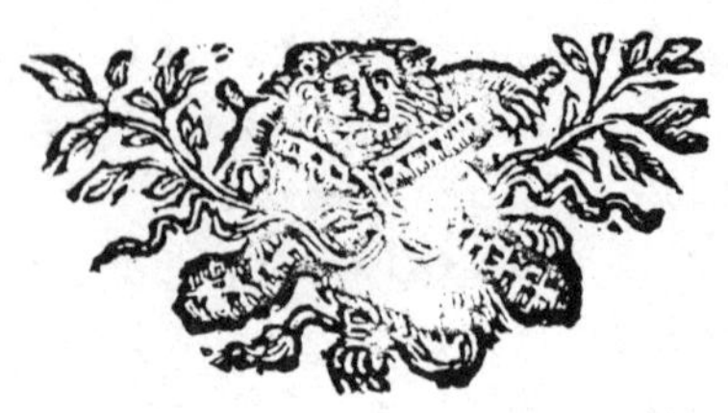

THE

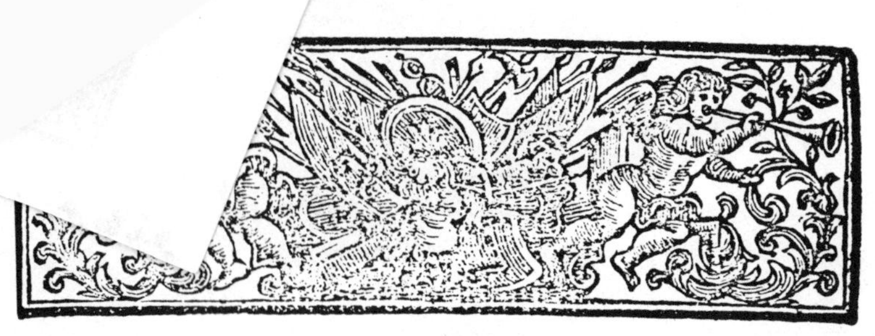

THE DISPENSARY.

CANTO I.

SPeak, Goddeſs! ſince 'tis Thou that beſt can'ſt tell,
How ancient Leagues to modern Diſcord fell;
And why Phyſicians were ſo cautious grown
Of Others Lives, and laviſh of their Own;
How by a Journey to th'*Elyſian* Plain
Peace triumph'd, and old Time return'd again.

Not far from that moſt celebrated Place,
Where angry * Juſtice ſhews her awful Face;
Where little Villians muſt ſubmit to Fate,
That great Ones may enjoy the World in State;
There ſtands a † Dome, Majeſtick to the Sight,
And ſumptuous Arches bear its oval Height;

* *Old Baily.* † *College of Phyſicians.*

A

A golden Globe plac'd high with artful Skill,
Seems, to the diſtant Sight, a gilded Pill:
This Pile was, by the Pious Patron's Aim,
Rais'd for a Uſe as Noble as its Frame:
Nor did the Learn'd Society decline
The Propagation of that great Deſign;
In all her Mazes, Nature's Face they view'd,
And as ſhe diſappear'd, their Search purſu'd.
Wrapt in the ſhades of Night the Goddeſs lies,
Yet to the learn'd unveils her dark Diſguiſe,
But ſhuns the groſs Acceſs of vulgar Eyes.

Now ſhe unfolds the faint, and dawning Strife
Of infant Atoms kindled into Life:
How ductile Matter new Meanders takes,
And ſlender Trains of twiſting Fibres makes.
And how the Viſcous ſeeks a cloſer Tone,
By juſt degrees to harden into Bone;
While the more Looſe flow from the vital Urn,
And in full Tides of Purple Streams return;
How lambent Flames from Life's bright Lamp ariſe,
And dart in Emanations through the Eyes;
How from each Sluice a gentle Torrent pours,
To ſlake a feav'riſh Heat with ambient Show'rs.
Whence, their Mechanick Pow'rs, the Spirits claim,
How great their Force, how delicate their Frame:
How the ſame Nerves are faſhion'd to ſuſtain
The greateſt Pleaſure and the greateſt Pain.
Why bileous Juice a Golden Light puts on,
And Floods of Chyle in Silver Currents run.
How the dim Speck of Entity began
T' extend its recent Form, and ſtretch to Man.

CANTO I.

To how minute an Origin we owe
Young *Ammon*, *Cæsar*, and the Great *Nassau*.
Why paler Looks impetuous Rage proclaim,
And why chill Virgins redden into Flame.
Why Envy oft transforms with wan Disguise,
And why gay Mirth sits smiling in the Eyes.
All Ice why *Lucrece*, or *Sempronia*, Fire,
Why *S----* rages to survive Desire.
Whence *Milo*'s Vigour at *Olympick*'s shown,
Whence Tropes to *F----* or Impudence to *S---*
How Matter, by the vary'd shape of Pores,
Or Idiots frames, or solemn Senators.

Hence 'tis we wait the wond'rous Cause to find,
How Body acts upon impassive Mind:
How Fumes of Wine the thinking Part can fire,
Past Hopes revive, and present Joys inspire:
Why our Complexions oft our Souls declare,
And how the Passions in the Features are:
How Touch and Harmony arise between
Corporeal Figure, and a Form unseen;
How quick their Faculties the Limbs fulfil,
And act at ev'ry Summons of the Will.
With mighty Truths, mysterious to descry,
Which in the Womb of distant Causes lye.

But now no grand Enquiries are descry'd,
Mean Faction reigns, where Knowledge should preside,
Feuds are encreas'd, and Learning laid aside.
Thus *Synods* oft, Concern for Faith conceal;
And for important *Nothings* shew a Zeal:

The

The drooping Sciences neglected pine,
And *Pæan*'s Beams with fading Lustre shine.
No Readers here with Hectick Looks are found,
Or Eyes in Rheum, thro' midnight-watchings, drown'd:
The lonely Edifice in Sweats complains
That nothing there but sullen Silence reigns.

This Place so fit for undisturb'd Repose,
The God of Sloth for his *Asylum* chose.
Upon a Couch of Down in these Abodes,
Supine with folded Arms he thoughtless nods;
Indulging Dreams his Godhead lull to Ease,
With Murmurs of soft Rills, and whisp'ring Trees.
The *Popyy* and each numbing Plant dispense
Their drowsy Virtue, and dull Indolence.
No Passions interrupt his easy Reign,
No Problems puzzle his Lethargick Brain,
But dark Oblivion guards his peaceful Bed,
And lazy Fogs hang ling'ring o'er his Head.

As at full length the pamper'd Monarch lay
Batt'ning in Ease, and slumb'ring Life away:
A spiteful Noise his downy Chains unties,
Hastes forward, and encreases as it flies.

First, some to cleave the stubborn * Flint engage,
Till urg'd by Blows, it sparkles into Rage:
Some temper Lute, some spacious Vessels move;
These Furnaces erect, and Those approve.

* *The Building of the Dispensary.*

Here

Here Phyals in nice Discipline are set,
There Gally-pots are rang'd in Alphabet.
In this place, Magazines of Pills you spy;
In that, like Forage, Herbs in Bundles lye.
While lifted Pestles brandish'd in the Air
Descend in Peals, and Civil Wars declare.
Loud Stroaks, with pounding Spice, the Fabrick rend,
And Aromatick Clouds in Spires ascend.

So when the *Cyclops* o'er their Anvils sweat,
And swelling Sinews ecchoing Blows repeat;
From the *Volcano*'s gross Eruptions rise,
And curling Sheets of Smoke obscure the Skies.

The slumb'ring God amaz'd at this new Din,
Thrice strove to rise, and thrice sunk down agen.
Listless he stretch'd, and gaping rubb'd his Eyes,
Then falter'd thus betwixt half Words and Sighs.

How impotent a Deity am I!
With Godhead born, but curs'd, that cannot die!
Thro' my Indulgence, Mortals hourly share
A grateful Negligence, and Ease from Care.
Lull'd in my Arms, how long have I with-held
The *Northern* Monarchs from the dusty Field.
How have I kept the *British* Fleet at Ease,
From tempting the rough Dangers of the Seas.
Hibernia owns the Mildness of my Reign,
And my Divinity's ador'd in *Spain*.
I Swains to *Sylvan* Solitudes convey,
Where stretch'd on Mossy Beds, they waste away,
In gentle Joys the Night, in Vows the Day.

What Marks of wond'rous Clemency I've ſhown,
Some Rev'rend *Worthies* of the Gown can own.
Triumphant Plenty, with a chearful Grace,
Basks in their Eyes, and ſparkles in their Face.
How ſleek their Looks, how goodly is their Mien,
When big they ſtrut behind a double Chin.
Each Faculty in Blandiſhments they lull,
Aſpiring to be venerably dull.
No learn'd Debates moleſt their downy Trance,
Or diſcompoſe their pompous Ignorance,
But undiſturb'd, they loiter Life away,
So wither Green, and bloſſom in Decay.
Deep ſunk in Down, they, by my gentle Care,
Avoid th' Inclemencies of Morning Air,
And leave to tatter'd * *Crape* the Drudgery of Pray'r.

Urim was civil, and not void of Senſe,
Had Humour, and a courteous Confidence.
So ſpruce he moves, ſo gracefully he cocks;
The hallow'd *Roſe* declares him Orthodox.
He paſs'd his eaſie Hours, inſtead of Pray'r,
In Madrigals, and *Philliſing* the Fair.
Conſtant at Feaſts, and each *Decorum* knew;
And ſoon as the *Deſſert* appear'd, withdrew.
Always obliging and without Offence,
And fancy'd for his gay Impertinence.
But ſee how ill miſtaken Parts ſucceed;
He threw off my Dominion, and would read;
Engag'd in Controverſie, wrangle well;
In *Convocation*-Language cou'd excel.

* *See Boil. Lutr.*

In

In Volumes prov'd the Church without Defence,
By nothing guarded but by *Providence* :
How Grace and Moderation diſagree ;
And Violence advances Charity.
Thus writ 'till none would read, becoming ſoon
A wretched Scribler, of a rare Buffoon.

Mankind my fond propitious Pow'r has try'd,
Too oft to own, too much to be deny'd.
And all I ask are Shades and ſilent Bow'rs,
To paſs in ſoft forgetfulneſs my Hours.
Oft have my Fears ſome diſtant *Villa* choſe,
O'er their *Quietus* where fat *Judges* doſe,
And lull their Cough and Conſcience to repoſe.
Or if ſome *Cloyſter*'s Refuge I implore,
Where holy *Drones* o'er dying Tapers ſnore:
The Peals of * *Naſſau*'s Arms theſe Eyes uncloſe,
Mine he moleſts, to give the World Repoſe.
That Eaſe I offer with Contempt He flies,
His Couch a Trench, his Canopy the Skies.
Nor Climes nor Seaſons his Reſolves controul,
Th' *Æquator* has no Heat, no Ice the *Pole*.
With Arms reſiſtleſs o'er the Globe he flies,
And leaves to *Jove* the Empire o' the Skies.

But as the ſlothful God to yawn begun,
He ſhook off the dull Miſt, and thus went on.

'Twas in this rev'rend Dome I ſought Repoſe,
Theſe Walls were that *Aſylum* I had choſe.

* *See Boil. Lut.*

Here have I rul'd long undisturb'd with Broils,
And laugh'd at Heroes, and their glorious Toils.
My Annals are in mouldy Mildews wrought,
With easie Insignificance of Thought.
But now some busie, enterprizing Brain
Invents new Fancies to renew my Pain,
And labours to dissolve my easie Reign.

With that, the God his darling *Phantom* calls,
And from his falt'ring Lips this Message falls:

Since Mortals will dispute my Pow'r, I'll try
Who has the greatest Empire, they or I.
Find *Envy* out, some Prince's Court attend,
Most likely there you'll meet the Famish'd Fiend.
Or where dull Criticks Author's Fate foretell;
Or where stale Maids or meager Eunuch's dwell.
Tell the bleak Fury what new Projects reign,
Among the Homicides of *Warwick-Lane*.
And what th' Event, unless she strait inclines
To blast their Hopes, and baffle their Designs.

More he had spoke, but suddain Vapours rise,
And with their silken Cords tie down his Eyes.

THE

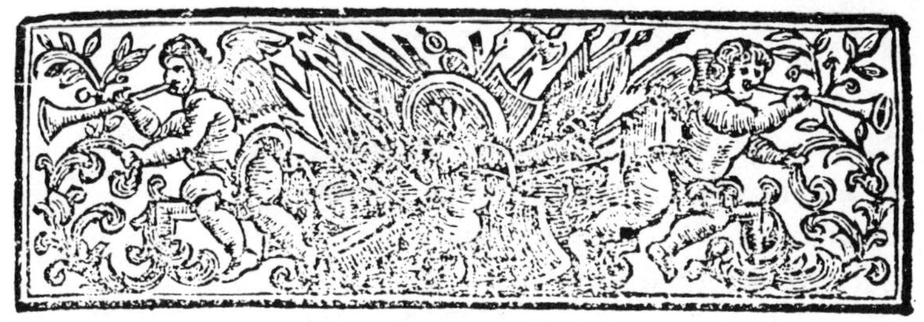

THE DISPENSARY.

CANTO II.

SOON as the Ev'ning veil'd the Mountains Heads,
And Winds lay hush'd in subterranean Beds;
Whilst sick'ning Flow'rs drink up the Silver Dew,
And *Beaus*, for some *Assembly*, dress anew;
The City Saints to Pray'rs and Play-house haste;
The Rich to Dinner, and the Poor to Rest:
Officious Phantom then prepar'd with Care
To slide on tender Pinions through the Air.
Oft he attempts the Summit of a Rock,
And oft the Hollow of some blasted Oak;
At length approaching where bleak *Envy* lay,
The hissing of her Snakes proclaim'd the way.

Beneath the gloomy Covert of an Yew,
That taints the Grass with sickly Sweats of Dew;

No verdant Beauty entertains the Sight,
But baneful Hemlock, and cold Aconite;
In a dark Grott the baleful Haggard lay,
Breathing black Vengeance, and infecting Day.
But how deform'd and worn with spiteful Woes,
When *Accius* has Applause, *Dorsennus* shows.
The cheerful Blood her meager Cheeks forsook,
And Basilisks sat Brooding in her Look;
A bald and bloated Toad-stool rais'd her Head;
The Plumes of boding Ravens were her Bed:
From her chapp'd Nostrils scalding Torrents fall,
And her sunk Eyes boil o'er in Floods of Gall.
Vulcano's labour thus with inward Pains,
Whilst Seas of melted Ore lay waste the Plains.

Around the Fiend in hideous Order sate
Foul bawling Infamy, and bold Debate:
Gruff Discontent, thro' Ignorance mis-led,
And clam'rous Faction at her Party's Head:
Restless Sedition still dissembling Fear,
And sly Hypocrisie with Pious Leer. *

Glouting with sullen Spight the Fury shook
Her clotter'd Locks, and blasted with each Look,
Then tore with canker'd Teeth the pregnant Scrolls,
Where Fame the Acts of Demi-Gods enrolls,
And as the rent Records in pieces fell,
Each Scrap did some Immortal Action tell.

This show'd, how fix'd as Fate *Torquatus* stood,
That, the fam'd Passage of the *Granick* Flood;

* *See* Dryd. *Fab.*

The

The *Julian* Eagles, here, their Wings display,
And there, like setting Stars, the *Decii* lay;
This does *Camillus* as a God extol,
That points at *Manlius* in the Capitol;
How *Cocbles* did the *Tyber*'s Surges brave,
How *Curtius* plung'd into the gaping Grave.
Great *Cyrus*, here, the *Medes* and *Persians* join,
And, there, th'immortal Battle of the *Boyn*.

As the light Messenger the Fury spy'd,
A while his crudling Blood forgot to glide:
Confusion on his fainting Vitals hung,
And falt'ring Accents flutter'd on his Tongue.
At length, assuming Courage, he convey'd
His Errand, then he shrunk into a Shade.

The Hag lay long revolving what might be
The blest Event of such an Embassie:
Then blazons in dread Smiles her hideous Form.
So Light'ning gilds the unrelenting Storm.
Thus she- - - -Mankind are blest, they riot still
Unbounded in Exorbitance of Ill.
By Devastation the rough Warrior gains,
And Farmers fatten most when Famine reigns;
For sickly Seasons the Physicians wait,
And Politicians thrive in Broils of State;
The Lover's easy when the Fair one sighs,
And Gods subsist not but by Sacrifice.

Each other Being some Indulgence knows;
Few are my Joys, but infinite my Woes.

My preſent Pain *Britannia*'s Genius wills,
And thus the Fates record my future Ills.

A Heroine ſhall *Albion*'s Scepter bear,
With Arms ſhall vanquiſh Earth, and Heav'n with Pray'r.
She on the World her Clemency ſhall ſhow'r,
And only to preſerve, exert her Pow'r.
Tyrants ſhall then their impious Aims forbear,
And *Blenheim*'s Thunder, more than * *Ætna*'s, fear.

Since by no Arts I therefore can defeat
The happy Enterprizes of the Great,
I'll calmly ſtoop to more inferior Things;
And try if my lov'd Snakes have Teeth or Stings.

She ſaid; and ſtrait ſhrill *Colon*'s Perſon took,
In Morals looſe, but moſt preciſe in Look,
Black-Fryars Annals lately pleas'd to call
Him Warden of *Apothecaries-Hall.*
And, when ſo dignify'd, did not forbear
That Operation which the Learn'd declare
Gives Cholicks eaſe, and makes the Ladies fair.
In trifling Show his Tinſel Talent lies,
And Form the want of Intellects ſupplies.
In Aſpect grand and goodly He appears,
Rever'd as Patriarchs in primæval Years.
Hourly his Learn'd Impertinence affords
A barren Superfluity of Words.
The Patient's Ears remorſeleſs he aſſails
Murthers with Jargon where his Med'cine fails.

* *In* Ætna *were forg'd the Thunder-bolts which* Jove *employ'd againſt the Ambition of the Giants.*

The

The Fury thus assuming *Colon*'s Grace,
So flung her Arms, so shuffl'd in her Pace.
Onward she hastens to the fam'd Abodes,
Where *Horoscope* invokes th' infernal Gods;
And reach'd the Mansion where the Vulgar run,
For Ruin throng, and pay to be undone.

This *Visionarie* various Projects tries,
And knows, that to be rich is to be Wise.
By useful Observations he can tell
The sacred Charms, that in true Sterling dwell.
How Gold makes a *Patrician* of a Slave,
A Dwarf an *Atlas*, a *Thersites* brave.
It cancels all Defects, and in their Place
Finds Sense in *Br*----, Charms in Lady *G*---*e*;
It guides the Fancy, and directs the Mind;
No Bankrupt ever found a Fair one kind.

So truly *Horoscope* its Virtue knows,
To this lov'd Idol 'tis, alone, he bows;
And fancies such bright Heraldry can prove,
The vile *Plebeian* but the third from *Jove*.

Long has he been of that amphibious Fry,
Bold to Prescribe, and busie to Apply.
His Shop the gazing Vulgar's Eyes employs
With Foreign Trinkets, and Domestick Toys.

Here, *Mummies* lay most reverendly stale,
And there, the *Tortoise* hung her Coat o' Mail;
Not far from some huge *Shark*'s devouring Head
The flying Fish their finny Pinnions spread.

Aloft

Aloft in Rows large Poppy Heads were ſtrung,
And near, a ſcaly Alligatur hung.
In this place, Drugs in muſty Heaps decay'd,
In that, dry'd Bladders, and drawn Teeth were laid.

An inner Room receives the num'rous Shoals,
Of ſuch as pay to be reputed Fools.
Globes ſtand by Globes, Volumes on Volumes lye,
And Planetary Schemes amuſe the Eye.
The Sage, in Velvet Chair, here lolls at Eaſe,
To promiſe future Health for preſent Fees.
Then, as from *Tripod*, ſolemn Shams reveals,
And what the Stars know nothing of, foretels.

One asks how ſoon *Panthea* may be won,
And longs to feel the Marriage Fetters on.
Others, convinc'd by melancholly Proof,
Enquire when curteous Fates will ſtrike 'em off.

Some, by what means they may redreſs the Wrong,
When Fathers the Poſſeſſion keep too long.
And ſome would know the Iſſue of their Cauſe,
And whether Gold can ſolder up its Flaws.
Poor pregnant *Lais* his Advice would have,
To looſe by Art what fruitful Nature gave:
And *Portia* old in expectation grown,
Laments her barren Curſe, and begs a Son.
Whilſt *Iris*, his Coſmetick *Waſh* would try,
To make her Bloom revive, and Lovers die.
Some ask for Charms, and others Philters chuſe,
To gain *Corinna*, and their Quartans loſe.

Young

Young *Hylas*, botch'd with Stains too foul to name,
In Cradle here renews his Youthful Frame:
Cloy'd with Desire, and surfeited with Charms,
A Hot-House he perfers to *Julia*'s Arms.
And old *Lucullus* wou'd th' *Arcanum* prove,
Of kindling in cold Veins the Sparks of Love.

Bleak Envy these dull Frauds with Pleasure sees,
And wonders at the senseless Mysteries.
In *Colon*'s Voice she thus calls out aloud
On *Horoscope* environ'd by the Crowd.

Forbear, forbear, thy vain Amusements cease,
Thy *Woodcocks* from their *Gines* a while release;
And to that dire Misfortune listen well,
Which thou shou'dst fear to know, or I to tell.
'Tis true, thou ever wast esteem'd by me
The great *Alcides* of our *Company*.
When we with Noble Scorn resolv'd to ease
Our selves from all Parochial Offices;
And to our Wealthier Patients left the Care,
And draggl'd Dignity of Scavenger:
Such Zeal in that Affair thou didst express,
Nought cou'd be equal, but the great Success.
Now call to Mind thy Gen'rous Prowess past,
Be what thou shou'dst, by thinking what thou wast:
The Faculty of *Warwick-Lane* Design,
If not to Storm, at least to Undermine.
Their Gates each Day Ten thousand Night-caps crowd,
And Mortars utter their Attempts aloud.
If they should once unmask our Mystery,
Each Nurse, ere long, wou'd be as learn'd as We;

Our

Our Art expos'd to ev'ry Vulgar Eye,
And none, in Complaisance to us, wou'd dye.
What if We claim their Right t' Assassinate,
Must they needs turn *Apothecaries* strait?
Prevent it, Gods! all Stratagems we try,
To crowd with new Inhabitants your Sky.
'Tis we who wait the Destinies Command,
To purge the troubled Air, and weed the Land.
And dare the *College* insolently aim
To equal our Fraternity in Fame?
Then let *Crabs* Eyes with *Pearl* for Virtue try,
Or *Highgate-Hill* with lofty *Pindus* vie:
So *Glo-worms* may compare with *Titan*'s Beams,
And *Hare-Court* Pump with *Aganippe*'s Streams.

Our Manufactures now they meanly sell,
And their true Value treacherously tell:
Nay, They discover too, (their spight is such,)
That Health, than Crowns more valu'd, costs not much.
Whilst we must steer our Conduct by these Rules,
To cheat as Tradesmen, or to starve as Fools.

At this fam'd *Horoscope* turn'd pale, and straight
In Silence tumbl'd from his Chair of State.
The Crowd in great Confusion sought the Door;
And left the *Magus* fainting on the Floor.
Whilst in his Breast the Fury breath'd a Storm,
Then sought her Cell, and reasum'd her Form.
Thus from the Sore altho' the Insect flies,
It leaves a Brood of Maggots in Disguise.

Officious

Officious *Squirt* in haste forsook his Shop,
To succour the expiring *Horoscope*.
Oft he essay'd the *Magus* to restore,
By Salt of *Succinum*'s prevailing Pow'r;
Yet still supine the solid Lumber lay
An Image of scarce animated Clay;
'Till Fates, indulgent when Disasters call,
By *Squirt*'s nice Hand apply'd a Urinal;
The Weight no sooner did the Steam receive,
But rous'd, and bless'd the stale Restorative.
The Springs of Life their former Vigour feel,
Such Zeal he had for that vile Utensil.

So when the great *Pelides*, *Thetis* found,
He knew the Sea-weed Scent, and th' Azure Goddess own'd.

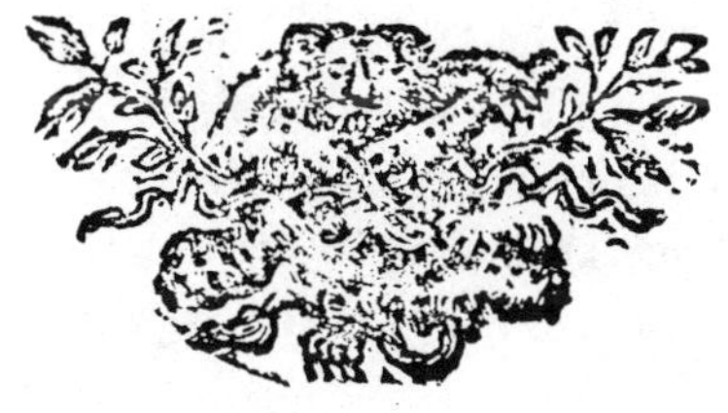

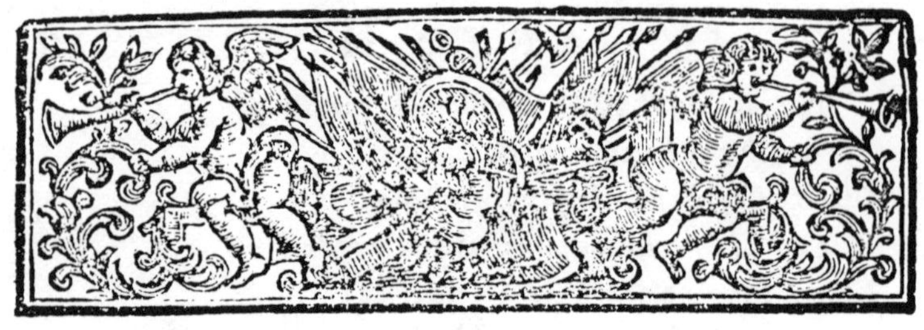

THE DISPENSARY.

CANTO III.

ALL Night the Sage in Pensive Tumults lay,
Complaining of the slow Approach of Day;
Oft turn'd him round, and strove to think no more
Of what shrill *Colon* said the Day before.
Cowslips and *Poppies* o'er his Eyes he spread,
And *S*- - - - - Works he laid beneath his Head.
But those blest Opiats still in vain he tries,
Sleep's gentle Image his Embraces flies.
Tumultuous Cares lay rolling in his Breast,
And thus his anxious Thoughts the Sage exprest.

Oft has this Planet roll'd around the Sun,
Since to consult the Skies, I first begun:
Such my Applause, so mighty my Success,
Some granted my Predictions more than Guess.

But

But, doubtful as I am, I'll entertain
This Faith, There can be no Miſtake in Gain.
For the dull World muſt Honour pay to thoſe
Who on their Underſtanding moſt impoſe.
Firſt Man creates, and then he fears the Elf,
Thus others cheat him not, but he himſelf;
He loaths the Subſtance, and he loves the Show;
You'll ne'er convince a Fool, Himſelf is ſo:
He hates Realities, and hugs the Cheat,
And ſtill the only Pleaſure's the Deceit.
So Meteors flatter with a dazling Dye
Which no Exiſtence has, but in the Eye.
At diſtance Proſpects pleaſe us, but when near,
We find but deſart Rocks, and fleeting Air.
From Stratagem to Stratagem we run,
And he knows moſt, who lateſt is undone.

Mankind one Day ſerene and free appear;
The next, they're cloudy, ſullen, and ſevere:
New Paſſions, new Opinions ſtill excite,
And what they like at Noon, they leave at Night.
They gain with Labour, what they quit with eaſe,
And Health, for want of Change, becomes Diſeaſe.
Religion's bright Authcrity they dare,
And yet are Slaves to Superſtitious Fear.
They Counſel others, but themſelves Deceive,
And tho' they're Cozen'd ſtill, they ſtill Believe.

So falſe their Cenſure, fickle their Eſteem,
This Hour they Worſhip; and the next Blaſpheme

Shall I then, who with penetrating Sight
Inſpect the Springs that guide each Appetite:
Who with unfathom'd Searches hourly pierce
The dark Receſſes of the Univerſe,
Be aw'd, if puny Emmets wou'd oppreſs;
Or fear their Fury, or their Name careſs?
If all the Fiends that in low Darkneſs reign,
Be not the Fictions of a ſickly Brain,
That Project, the * *Diſpenſary* they call,
Before the Moon can blunt her Horns, ſhall fall.

With that, a Glance from mild *Aurora*'s Eyes
Shoots thro' the Chryſtal Kingdoms of the Skies;
The Savage Kind in Foreſts ceaſe to roam,
And Sots o'ercharg'd with nauſeous Loads reel home.
Drums, Trumpets, Haut-boys wake the ſlumbering Pair;
Whilſt Bridegroom ſighs, and thinks the Bride leſs fair.
Light's chearful Smiles o'er th' Azure Waſte are ſpread,
And Miſs from Inns o'Court bolts out unpaid.
The Sage tranſported at th'approaching Hour,
Imperiouſly thrice thunder'd on the Floor;
Officious *Squirt* that Moment had acceſs,
His Truſt was great, his Vigilance no leſs.
To him thus *Horoſcope*,

My kind Companion in this dire Affair,
Which is more light, ſince you aſſume a Share;
Fly with what haſte you us'd to do of old,
When *Clyſter* was in danger to be cold:
With Expedition on the Beadle call,
To ſummon all the *Company* to th'*Hall*.

* *Medicines made up there, for the uſe of the Poor.*

Away the friendly Coadjutor flies.
Swift as from Phyal Steams of *Harts-horn* riſe.
The *Magus* in the int'rim mumbles o'er
Vile Terms of Art to ſome Infernal Pow'r,
And draws Myſterious Circles on the Floor.
But from the gloomy Vault no glaring Spright
Aſcends, to blaſt the tender Bloom of Light.
No myſtick Sounds from *Hell*'s deteſted Womb,
In dusky Exhalations upwards come.
And now to raiſe an Altar He decrees,
To that devouring Harpy call'd *Diſeaſe*:
Then Flow'rs in Caniſters he haſtes to bring,
The wither'd Product of a blighted Spring.
With cold *Solanum* from the *Pontick* Shore,
The Roots of *Mandrake* and black *Ellebore*,
The Griper *Senna*, and the Puker *Rue*,
The Sweetner *Saſſafras* are added too;
And on the Structure next he heaps a load
Of *Sulpher*, *Turpentine* and *Maſtick* Wood:
Gums, Foſſiles too the Pyramid increas'd.
A *Mummy* next, once Monarch of the Eaſt.
Then from the Compter he takes down the File,
And with Preſcriptions lights the ſolemn Pile.

Feebly the Flames on clumſie Wings aſpire,
And ſmoth'ring Fogs of Smoke benight the Fire.
With ſorrow he beheld the ſad Portent,
Then to the Hag theſe *Orizons* he ſent.

Diſeaſe! thou ever moſt propitious Pow'r,
Whoſe kind Indulgence we diſcern each Hour:

Thou well canſt boaſt thy num'rous Pedigree
Begot by Sloth, maintain'd by Luxury.
In gilded Palaces thy Prowefs reigns,
But flies the humble Sheds of Cottage Swains.
To You ſuch Might and Energy belong,
You nip the Blooming, and unnerve the Strong.
The Purple Conqueror in Chains you bind,
And are to us your Vaſſals only kind.

If, in return, all Diligence we pay
To fix your Empire, and confirm your Sway,
Far as the weekly Bills can reach around,
From *Kent-ſtreet* End to fam'd St. *Giles*'s-*Pound*;
Behold this poor Libation with a Smile,
And let auſpicious Light break through the Pile.

He ſpoke; and on the Pyramid he laid
Bay Leaves and Vipers Hearts, and thus he ſaid;
As *Theſe* conſume in this myſterious Fire,
So let the curs'd *Diſpenſary* * expire
And as *Thoſe* crackle in the Flames, and die,
So let its Veſſels burſt, and Glaſſes fly.
But a ſiniſter Cricket ſtrait was heard,
The Altar fell, the Off'ring diſappear'd.
As the fam'd Wight the Omen did regret,
Squirt brought the News the *Company* was met.

Nigh where *Fleet-Ditch* deſcends in ſable Streams,
To waſh his ſooty *Naiads* in the *Thames*;
There ſtands a † Structure on a riſing Hill,
Where *Tyro*'s take their Freedom out to kill.

* *See the Alluſion. Theoc. Pharm.* † *Apothecaries Hall.*

Some

Some Pictures in these dreadful Shambles tell,
How by the *Delian* God, the *Pithon* fell;
And how *Medea* did the *Philter* brew,
That cou'd in *Æson*'s Veins young Force renew,
How mournful * *Myrrha* for her Crimes appears,
And heals hysterick Matrons still with Tears.
How *Mentha* and *Althea*, Nymphs no more,
Revive in sacred Plants, and Health restore.
How sanguine Swains their am'rous Hours repent,
When Pleasure's past, and Pains are permanent;
And how frail Nymphs, oft by Abortion, aim
To lose a Substance, to preserve a Name.

Soon as each Member in his Rank was plac'd,
Th' Assembly *Diasenna* thus address'd.

My kind Confederates, if my poor Intent,
As 'tis sincere, had been but prevalent,
We here had met on some more safe Design,
And on no other Bus'ness but to Dine;
The *Faculty* had still maintain'd their Sway,
And Int'rest then had bid us but obey;
This only Emulation we had known,
Who best cou'd fill his Purse, and thin the Town.
But now from gath'ring Clouds Destruction pours,
Which ruins with mad Rage our *Halcyon* Hours:
Mists from black Jealousies the Tempest form,
Whilst late Divisions reinforce the Storm.
Know, when these Feuds, like those at Law, are past,
The Winners will be Losers at the last.

* *See Ov. Met.*

Like

Like Heroes in Sea-Fights we ſeek Renown,
To fire ſome Hoſtile Ship, we burn our own.
Who-e'er throws Duſt againſt the Wind, deſcries
He throws it, in effect, but in his Eyes.
That Juggler which another's Slight will ſhow,
But teaches how the World his own may know.

Thrice happy were thoſe golden Days of old,
When dear as *Burgundy*, *Ptiſans* were ſold;
When Patients choſe to die with better Will,
Than breathe, and pay th'*Apothecary*'s Bill.
And cheaper than for our Aſſiſtance call,
Might go to *Aix* or *Bourbon*, Spring and Fall.

Then Prieſts increas'd, and Piety decay'd,
Churchmen the Church's Purity betray'd;
Their Lives and Doctrine, Slaves and Atheiſts made.
The Laws were but the hireling Judge's Senſe;
Juries were ſway'd by venal Evidence.
Fools were promoted to the Council-Board,
Tools to the Bench, and Bullies to the Sword.
Penſions in Private were the Senate's Aim;
And Patriots for a Place abandon'd Fame.

But now no influencing Art remains,
For *S----rs* has the Seal, and *Naſſau* reigns.
And we, in ſpight of our Reſolves, muſt bow,
And ſuffer by a Reformation too.
For now late Jars our Practices detect,
And Mines, when once Diſcover'd loſe Effect.
Diſſentions, like ſmall Streams, are firſt begun,
Scarce ſeen they riſe, but gather as they run:

So

So Lines that from their Parallel decline,
More they proceed, the more they ſtill diſ-join.
'Tis therefore my Advice, in haſte we ſend,
And beg the *Faculty* to be our Friend;
Send ſwarms of Patients, and our Quarrels end.
So awful *Beadles*, if the *Vagrant* treat,
Strait turn familiar, and their *Faſces* quit.
In vain we but contend, that Planet's Pow'r
Thoſe Vapours can diſperſe it rais'd before.

As he prepar'd the Miſchief to recite,
Keen *Colorynthis* paus'd and foam'd with Spight.
Sow'r Ferments on his ſhining Surface ſwim,
Work up to Froth, and bubble o'er the Brim:
Not *Beauties* fret ſo much if Frecles come,
Or Noſe ſhou'd redden in the Drawing-Room;
Or *Lovers* that miſtake th' appointed Hour,
Or in the lucky Minute want the Pow'r.

Thus He- - - -Thou Scandal of great *Pæan*'s Art.
At thy Approach the Springs of Nature ſtart,
The Nerves unbrace: Nay at the Sight of thee,
A Scratch turns Cancer, Itch a Leproſie.
Coud'ſt Thou propoſe, That we, the *Friends* o'Fates,
Who fill *Church-yards*, and who unpeople States,
Who baffle Nature, and diſpoſe of Lives,
Whilſt *Ruſſel*, as we pleaſe, or ſtarves, or thrives,
Shou'd e'er ſubmit to their deſpotick Will,
Who out o'Conſultation ſcarce can kill?
The tow'ring *Alps* ſhall ſooner ſink to Vales,
And *Leaches*, in our Glaſſes, ſwell to *Whales*;

Or

Or *Norwich* trade in Implements of Steel,
And *Bromingham* in Stuffs and Druggets deal!
Allys at *Wapping* furnish us new Modes,
And *Monmouth-street*, *Versailles* with Riding-hoods;
The Sick to th'*Hundreds* in pale Throngs repair,
And change the *Gravel-Pits* for *Kentish* Air.
Our Properties must on our Arms depend;
'Tis next to Conquer, bravely to Defend.
'Tis to the Vulgar, Death too harsh appears;
The Ill we feel is only in our Fears.

To Die, is Landing on some silent Shoar,
Where Billows never break nor Tempests roar:
E'er well we feel the friendly Stroke, 'tis o'er.
The Wise thro' thought th' Insults of Death defy;
The Fools, thro' bless'd Insensibility
'Tis what the Guilty fear, the Pious crave;
Sought by the Wretch, and vanquish'd by the Brave.
It eases Lovers, sets the Captive free;
And, tho' a Tyrant, offers Liberty.

Sound but to Arms, the Foe shall soon confess
Our Force encreases, as our Funds grow less;
And what requir'd such Industry to raise,
We'll scatter into nothing as we please.
Thus they'll acknowledge, to Annihilate
Shews no less wond'rous Pow'r than to Create.
We'll raise our num'rous Cohorts, and oppose
The feeble Forces of our pigmy Foes;
Legions of Quacks shall join us on the Place,
From Great *Kirleus* down to *Doctor Case*.

Tho

Tho' ſuch vile Rubbiſh ſink, yet we ſhall riſe;
Directors ſtill ſecure the greateſt Prize.
Such poor Supports ſerve only like a Stay;
The Tree once fix'd, its *Reſt* is torn away.

So Patriots, in the time of Peace and Eaſe,
Forget the Fury of the late Diſeaſe:
On Dangers paſt, ſerenely think no more;
And curſe the Hand that heal'd the Wound before.

Arm therefore gallant Friends, 'tis Honour's Call,
Or let us boldly Fight, or bravely Fall.

To this the *Seſſion* ſeem'd to give Conſent,
Much lik'd the War, but dreaded much th'Event.
At length the growing Diff'rence to compoſe,
Two Brothers, nam'd *Aſcarides* aroſe.
Both had the Volubility of Tongue,
In Meaning faint, but in Opinion ſtrong.
To ſpeak they both aſſum'd a like Pretence,
The Elder gain'd his juſt Pre-eminence;

Thus he: 'Tis true, when Priviledge and Right
Are once invaded, Honour bids us Fight.
But e'er we once engage in Honour's Cauſe,
Firſt know what Honour is, and whence it was.

Scorn'd by the Baſe, 'tis courted by the Brave,
The Heroe's Tyrant, and the Coward's Slave.
Born in the noiſie Camp, it lives on Air;
And both exiſts by Hope and by Deſpair.

Angry

Angry when e'er a Moment's Eaſe we gain,
And reconcil'd at our Returns of Pain.
It lives, when in Death's Arms the Heroe lies,
But when his Safety he conſults it dies.
Bigotted to this Idol, we diſclaim
Reſt, Health, and Eaſe, for nothing but a Name.

Then let us, to the Field before we move,
Know, if the Gods our Enterprize approve.
Suppoſe th'unthinking Faculty unveil
What we, thro' wiſer Conduct, wou'd conceal:
Is't Reaſon we ſhou'd quarrel with the Glaſs
That ſhews the monſtrous Features of our Face?
Or grant ſome grave Pretenders have of late
Thought fit an Innovation to create;
Soon they'll repent, what raſhly they begun:
Tho' Projects pleaſe, Projectors are undone.
All Novelties muſt this Succeſs expect,
When good, our Envy; and when bad, Neglect:
If Reaſon cou'd direct, e'er now each Gate
Had born ſome Trophy of Triumphal State.
Temples had told how *Greece* and *Belgia* owe
Troy and *Namur* to *Jove* and to *Naſſau*.

Then ſince no Veneration is allow'd,
Or to the real, or th' appearing Good;
The Project that we vainly apprehend,
Muſt as it blindly roſe, as vilely end.
Some Members of the Faculty there are,
Who Int'reſt prudently to Oaths prefer.
Our Friendſhip with vain Airs they poorly court,
And boaſt their Politicks are our Support.

Them

Them we'll consult about this Enterprize,
And boldly Execute what they Advise.

But from below (while such Resolves they took)
Some *Aurum Fulminans* the * Fabrick shook.
The Champions, daunted at the Crack, retreat,
Regard their Safety, and their Rage forget.

So when at *Bathos* Earth's big Offspring strove
To scale the Skies, and wage a War with *Jove*;
Soon as the *Ass* of old *Silenus* bray'd,
The trembling Rebels in Confusion fled.

* *The Room the Apothecaries meet in, is over the Laboratory.*

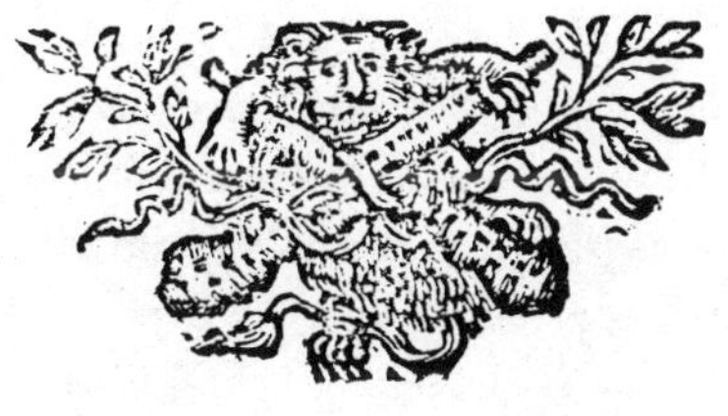

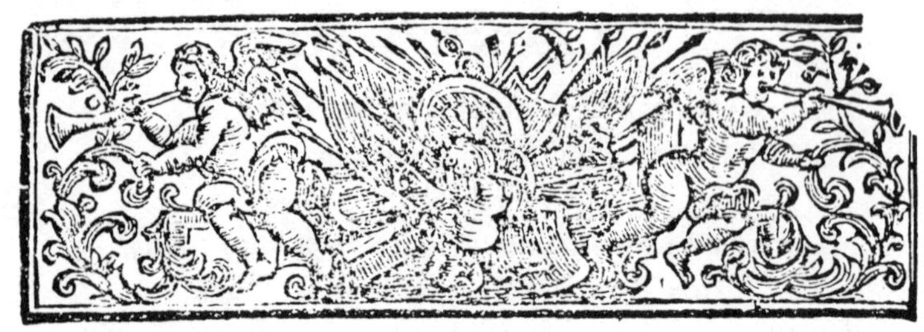

THE DISPENSARY.

CANTO IV.

NOT far from that frequented Theatre,
Where wand'ring Punks each Night at Five repair;
Where Purple Emperors in Buskins tread,
And rule imaginary Worlds for Bread;
Where *Bently* by old Writers, wealthy grew,
And *Briscoe* lately was undone by New,
There triumphs a *Physician* of Renown,
To none but such as rust in Health unknown.
None e'er was plac'd more fitly to impart
His known Experience, and his healing Art.
When *Bur------ss* deafens all the list'ning Press
With Peals of most Seraphick Emptiness;
Or when Mysterious F-----*n* mounts on high,
To preach his Parish to a Lethargy:
This *Æsculapis* waits hard by, to ease
The *Martyrs* of such Christian Cruelties.

Long

Long has this darling Quarter of the Town,
For Lewdness, Wit, and Gallantry been known.
All sorts meet here, of whatsoe'er Degree,
To blend and justle into Harmony.
The Criticks each advent'rous Author scan,
And praise or censure as They like the Man.
The Weeds of Writings for the Flowers they cull;
So nicely Tasteless, so correctly Dull!
The Politicians of *Parnassus* prate,
And Poets canvass the Affairs of State;
The Cits ne'er talk of Trade and Stock, but tell
How *Virgil* writ, how bravely *Turnus* fell.
The Country-Dames drive to *Hippolito*'s,
First find a Spark, and after lose a Nose.
The Lawyer for Lac'd Coat the Robe does quit,
He grows a Madman, and then turns a Wit.
And in the Cloister pensive *Strephon* waits,
'Till *Chloe*'s Hackney comes, and then retreats;
And if th'ungenerous Nymph a Shaft lets fly
More fatally than from a sparkling Eye,
Mirmillo, that fam'd *Opifer*, is nigh.

The trading Tribe oft thither throng to Dine,
And want of Elbow-room supply in Wine.
Cloy'd with Variety, they surfeit there,
Whilst the wan Patients on thin Gruel fare.
'Twas here the Champions of the Party met,
Of their Heroick Enterprize to treat.
Each Heroe a tremendous Air put on,
And stern *Mirmillo* in these Words begun:

'Tis with concern, my Friends, I meet you here;
No Grievance you can know, but I must share.
'Tis plain, my Int'rest you've advanc'd so long,
Each Fee, tho' I was mute, wou'd find a Tongue.
And in return, tho' I have strove to rend
Those Statutes, which on Oath I should defend;
Such Arts are Trifles to a gen'rous Mind:
Great Services, as great Returns shou'd find.
And you'll perceive, this Hand, when Glory calls,
Can brandish Arms as well as Urinals.

Oxford and all her passing Bells can tell,
By this Right Arm what mighty Numbers fell,
Whilst others meanly ask'd whole Months to slay,
I oft dispatch'd the Patient in a Day;
With Pen in Hand I push'd to that Degree,
I scacre had left a Wretch to give a Fee.
Some fell by *Laudanum*, and some by *Steel*,
And Death in Ambush lay in ev'ry Pill.
For save or slay this Privilege we claim,
Tho Credit suffers, the Reward's the same.

What tho' the Art of Healing we pretend
He that designs it least, is most a Friend.
Into the right we err, and must confess
To oversights we often owe success.
Thus *Bessus* got the Battle in the *Play*,
His glorious Cowardise restor'd the Day.
So the fam'd *Grecian* Piece ow'd its Desert
To chance, and not the labour'd Stroaks of Art.

Physi-

Physicians if they're wise shou'd never think
Of any Arms but such as Pen and Ink:
But th' Enemy, at their Expence shall find,
When Honour calls, I'll scorn to stay behind.

He said; and seal'd th' Engagement with a Kiss,
Which was return'd by younger *Askaris*;
Who thus advanc'd: Each Word, Sir, you impart,
Has something killing in it, like your Art.
How much we to your boundless Friendship owe,
Our Files can speak, and your Prescriptions show.
Your Ink descends in such Excessive Show'rs,
'Tis plain, you can regard no Health but ours.
Whilst poor Pretenders puzzle o'er a Case,
You but appear, and give the *Coup de Grace*..
O that near * *Xanthus* Banks you had but dwelt,
When *Ilium* first *Achaian* Fury felt,
The horned River then had curs'd in vain
Young *Peleus*' Arm, that choak'd his Stream with Slain
No Trophies you had left for *Greeks* to raise,
Their Ten Years Toil, you'd finish'd in Ten Days.
Fate smiles on your attempts, and when you list,
In vain the Cowards fly, or Brave resist,
Then let us Arm, we need not fear success;
No Labours are too hard for *Hercules*.
Our Military Ensigns we'll display;
Conquest pursues, where Courage leads the Way,

To this design shrill *Querpo* did agree
A zealous Member of the *Faculty*;

**See Hom. Il.*

His Sire's pretended pious Steps he treads,
And where the Doctor fails, the Saint succeeds.
A Conventicle flesh'd his greener Years,
And his full Age the righteous Rancour shares,
Thus Boys hatch Game-Eggs under Birds o'prey,
To make the Fowl more furious for the Fray.

Slow *Carus* next discover'd his Intent,
With painful Pauses mutt'ring what he meant,
His Sparks of Life in spight of Drugs retreat,
So cold, that only *Calentures* can heat,
In his chill Veins the sluggish Puddle flows.
And loads with lazy Fogs his sable Brows.
Legions of Lunaticks about him press,
His Province is lost Reason to redress.
So when perfumes their fragrant Scent give o'er,
Nought can their Odour, like a Jakes, restore.
When for Advice the Vulgar throng, he's found
With Lumber of vile Books besieg'd around.
The gazing Throng acknowledge their Surprize,
And deaf to Reason, still consult their Eyes.
Well he perceives, the World will often find,
To catch the Eye, is to convince the Mind,
Thus a weak State, by wise distrust enclines
To num'rous Stores, and Strength in Magazines.
So Fools are always most profuse of Words,
And Cowards never fail of longest Swords.
Abandon'd Authors here a refuge meet,
And from the World, to Dust and Worms retreat.
Here Dregs and Sediment of Auctions reign.
Refuse of Fairs, and Gleanings of *Duck-Lane*.

And

And up these Walls much *Gothick* Lumber climbs,
With *Swiss* Philosophy, and *Runick* Rhimes.
Hither, retriev'd from *Cooks* and *Grocers*, come
M---- Works entire, and endless Reams of *Bl*----*m*.
Where would the long neglected *C*---*s* fly,
If bounteous *Carus* shou'd refuse to buy?
But each vile Scribler's happy on this Score,
He'll find some *Carus* still to read him o're.

Nor must we the obsequious *Umbra* spare,
Who soft by Nature, yet declar'd for War.
But when some Rival Pow'r invades a Right,
Flies set on Flies, and Turtles Turtles fight.
Else Courteous *Umbra* to the last had been
Demurely meek, insipidly serene.
With him, the Present still some Virtues have,
The vain are sprightly, and the stupid, grave;
The Slothful, negligent; the Foppish, neat;
The Lewd are airy; and the Sly, discreet.
A Wren an Eagle, a Baboon a Beau;
C---- a *Lycurgus*, and a *Phocion*, R----

Heroick Ardour now th' Assembly warms,
Each Combatant breaths nothing but Alarms.
For future Glory, while the Scheme is laid,
Fam'd *Horoscope* thus offers to dissuade;

Since of each Enterprize th' Event's unknown,
We'll quit the Sword, and hearken to the Gown.

---

* *See the Imitation, Hor. Stat. the 3d.*

Nigh

Nigh lives *Vagellius*, one reputed long
For Strength of Lungs, and Pliancy of Tongue.
For Fees, to any Form he moulds a Cause,
The Worst has Merits, and the Best has Flaws.
Five Guineas make a Criminal to Day,
And ten to Morrow wipe the Stain away.
Whatever he affirms is undeny'd,
Milo's the Lecher, *Clodius* th'Homicide.
Cato pernicious, *Catiline* a Saint,
Or-----d suspected, *D----b* innocent.
To Law then Friends, for 'tis by Fate decreed,
Vagellius, and our Money, shall succeed.
Know; when I first invok'd *Disease* by Charms
To prove propitious to our future Arms;
Ill Omens did the Sacrifice attend,
Nor wou'd the *Sybil* from her *Grott* ascend.

As *Horoscope* urg'd farther to be heard,
He thus was interrupted by a *Bard*;

In vain your Magick Mysteries you use,
Such Sounds the *Sybil*'s sacred Ears abuse.
These Lines the pale Divinity shall raise,
Such is the Pow'r of Sound, and Force of Lays.

Arms meet with Arms, Fauchions with Fauchions clash,
And sparks of Fire struck out from Armour flash.
Thick Clouds of Dust contending Warriors raise,
And hideous War o'er all the Region brays.
Some raging ran with huge Herculean *Clubs,*
Some massy Balls of Brass, some mighty Tubs
Of Cynders bore.------

Naked

Naked and half-burnt Hills with hideous Wreck
Affright the Skies, and fry the Ocean's Back.

As he went rumbling on, the *Fury* strait
Crawl'd in, her Limbs cou'd scarce support the Weight.
A ruful Rag her meager Forehead bound,
And faintly her furr'd Lips these Accents found.

Mortal, how dar'st thou with such Lines address
My awful Seat, and trouble my Recess?
In *Essex* Marshy Hundreds is a Cell,
Where lazy Fogs, and drisling Vapours dwell:
Thither raw Damps on drooping Wings repair,
And shiv'ring Quartanes shake the sickly Air.
There, when fatigu'd, some silent Hours I pass,
And substitute Physicians in my Place.
Then dare not, for the future, once rehearse
The Dissonance of such untuneful Verse.
But in your Lines let Energy be found,
And learn to rise in Sense, and sink in Sound.
Harsh Words, tho' pertinent, uncouth appear;
None please the Fancy, who offend the Ear.
In Sense and Numbers if you would excel,
Read *W-----*, consider *D-----n* well.
In one, what vig'rous Turns of Fancy shine,
In th'other, *Syrens* warble in each Line.
If *D-----*'s sprightly Muse but touch the Lyre,
The *Smiles* and *Graces* melt in soft Desire,
And little *Loves* confess their am'rous Fire.
The gentle *Isis* claims the Ivy Crown,
To bind th'immortal Brows of *A-----n*.

As

As tuneful *C----ve* tries his rural Strains,
Pan quits the Woods, the list'ning Fawns the Plains;
And *Philomel*, in Notes like his, complains.
And *Britain*, since *Pausanias* was writ,
Knows *Spartan* Virtue, and *Athenian* Wit.
When *St-----* paints the Godlike Acts of Kings,
Or, what *Apollo* dictates, *P-----* sings,
The Banks of *Rhine* a pleas'd Attention show,
And Silver *Sequana* forgets to flow.

Such just Examples carefully read o'er,
Slide without falling, without straining, soar.
Oft tho' your Stroaks surprize, you shou'd not chuse
A Theme so mighty for a Virgin Muse.
Long did * *Apelles* his fam'd Piece decline,
His *Alexander* was his last Design.
'Tis *M------ue*'s rich Vein alone must prove,
None but a *Phidias* should attempt a *Jove*.

The Fury paus'd, 'till with a frightful Sound
A rising Whirlwind burst the unhallow'd Ground.
Then she------ The Deity we *Fortune* call,
Tho' distant rules and influences all.
Strait for her Favour to her Court repair,
Important Embassies ask Wings of Air.

Each wond'ring stood, but *Horoscope*'s great Soul
That Dangers ne'er alarm, nor Doubts controul;
Rais'd on the Pinions of the bounding Wind,
Out-flew the Rack, and left the Hours behind.

* *See Hor. B. 2. Ep. 1. Plin. Plut. Cic. Ep. Val. Max.*

The

The Ev'ning now with Bluſhes warms the Air,
The Steer reſigns the Yoke, the Hind his Care.
The Clouds above with golden Edgings glow,
And falling Dews refreſh the Earth below.
The Bat with ſooty Wings flits thro' the Grove,
The Reeds ſcarce ruſtle, nor the Aſpine move,
And all the feather'd Folks forbear their Lays of Love,
Thro' the tranſparent Region of the Skies,
Swift as a Wiſh the Miſſionary flies,
With wonder he ſurveys the upper Air,
And the gay gilded Meteors ſporting there.
How lambent Jellies kind'ling in the Night,
Shoot thro' the *Æther* in a Trail of Light;
How riſing Steams in th'azure Fluid blend,
Or fleet in Clouds, or in ſoft Show'rs deſcend;
Or if the ſtubborn Rage of Cold prevail,
In Flakes they fly, or fall in moulded Hail.
How Hony Dews embalm the fragrant Morn,
And the fair Oak with luſcious Sweats adorn.
How Heat and Moiſture mingle in a Maſs,
Or belch in Thunder, or in Light'ning blaze.
Why nimble Coruſcations ſtrike the Eye,
And bold *Tornado*'s bluſter in the Sky.
Why a prolifick *Aura* upward tends,
Ferments, and in a living Show'r deſcends.
How Vapours hanging on the tow'ring Hills
In Breezes ſigh, or weep in warbling Rills:
Whence Infant Winds their tender Pinions try,
And River Gods their thirſty Urns ſupply.

The

The wond'ring Sage pursues his airy Flight,
And braves the chill unwholsome Damps of Night;
He views the Tracts where Luminaries rove,
To settle Seasons here, and Fates above.
The bleak *Arcturus* still forbid the Seas,
The stormy *Kidds*, the weeping *Hyades*:
The shining * *Lyre* with Strains attracting more
Heav'ns glitt'ring Mansions now than † Hell's before.
Glad *Cassiopeia* circling in the Sky,
And each brave *Churchil* of the Galaxy.

Aurora on *Etesian* Breezes born,
With blushing Lips breaths out the sprightly Morn;
Each Flow'r in Dew their short-liv'd Empire weeps,
And *Cynthia* with her lov'd *Endymion* sleeps.
As through the Gloom the *Magus* cuts his Way,
Imperfect Objects tell the doutful Day.
Dim he discerns Majestick *Atlas* rise,
And bend beneath the Burthen of the Skies.
His tow'ring Brows aloft no Tempests know,
Whilst Light'ning flies, and Thunder rolls below.

Distant from hence beyond a Waste of Plains,
Proud *Teneriff* his Giant Brother reigns;
With breathing Fire his pitchy Nostrils glow,
As from his Sides he shakes the fleecy Snow.
Around this hoary Prince, from wat'ry Beds,
His Subject Islands raise their verdant Heads;
The Waves so gently wash each rising Hill,
The Land seems floating, and the Ocean still.

* Orpheus's *Harp made a Constellation*,

† *See* Manil.

Eternal

Eternal Spring with ſmiling Verdure here
Warms the mild Air, and crowns the youthful Year.
From Cryſtal Rocks tranſparent Riv'lets flow;
The Tub'roſe ever breathes, and Violets blow.
The Vine undreſs'd her ſwelling Cluſters bears,
The lab'ring Hind the mellow Olive cheers;
Bloſſoms and Fruit at once the * Citron ſhows,
And as ſhe pays, diſcovers ſtill ſhe owes.
The Orange to the Sun her Pride diſplays,
And gilds her fragrant Apples with his Rays.
No Blaſts e'er diſcompoſe the peaceful Sky,
The Springs but murmur, and the Winds but ſigh.
The tuneful Swans on gliding Rivers float,
And warbling Dirges, die on ev'ry Note.
Where *Flora* treads her *Zephyr* Garlands flings,
And ſcatters Odours from his Purple Wings;
Whilſt Birds from Woodbine Bow'rs and Jeſmine Groves
Chaunt their glad Nuptials, and unenvy'd Loves.
Mild Seaſons, riſing Hills, and ſilent Dales,
Cool Grotto's, Silver Brooks, and flow'ry Vales,
Groves fill'd with balmy Shrubs in pomp appear,
And ſcent with Gales of Sweets the circling Year.

These happy Iſles, where endleſs Pleaſures wait,
Are ſtil'd by tuneful Bards - - - - The *Fortunate*.
On high, where no hoarſe Winds nor Clouds reſort,
The hoodwink'd Goddeſs keeps her partial Court.
Upon a Wheel of † *Amethyſt* ſhe ſits,
Gives and reſumes, and ſmiles and frowns by Fits.

* Wall. † *This Stone reckon'd fortunate; ſee the Hiſt. of Nat. Magick.*

In this ſtill Labyrinth, around her lye
Spells, Philters, Globes, and Schemes of Palmiſtry:
A *Sigil* in this Hand the *Gypſie* bears,
In th'other a prophetick Sive and Sheers.

The Dame by Divination knew, that ſoon
The *Magus* wou'd appear-----and then begun
Hail, ſacred Seer! thy Embaſſie I know,
Wars muſt enſue, the Fates will have it ſo.
Dread Feats ſhall follow, and Diſaſters great,
* Pills charge on Pills, and Bolus Bolus meet:
Both Sides ſhall conquer, and yet Both ſhall fail;
The Mortar now, and then the Urinal.

To thee alone my Influence I owe;
Where Nature has deny'd, my Favours flow.
'Tis I that give (ſo mighty is my Pow'r)
Faith to the *Jew*, Complexion to the *Moor*.
I am the Wretch's Wiſh, the *Rook*'s Pretence,
The Sluggard's Eaſe, the Coxcomb's Providence.
Sir *Scrape-Quill*, once a ſupple ſmiling Slave,
Looks lofty now, and inſolently Grave;
Builds, Settles, Purchaſes, and has each Hour
Caps from the Rich, and Curſes from the Poor.
Spadillio, that at Table ſerv'd o' late,
Drinks rich Tockay himſelf, and eats in Plate;
Has *Levees*, *Villas*, Miſtreſſes in ſtore,
And owns the Racers which he rubb'd before.

Souls heav'nly born my faithleſs Boons deſy;
The Brave is to himſelf a Deity.

* *See the Alluſion*, Lucan.

Tho'

Tho' bleſt *Aſtrea*'s gone, ſome Soil remains
Where Fortune is the Slave, and Merit reigns,

The *Tyber* boaſts his *Julian* Progeny,
Thames his *Naſſau*, the *Nyle* his *Ptolomy*.
Iberia, yet for future Sway deſign'd,
Shall, for a *H - - - -*, a greater *M - - - -* find.
Thus * *Ariadne* in proud Triumph rode,
She loſt a † Heroe, and ſhe found a ‖ God.

* *See Steph.* † Theſeus. ‖ Bacchus.

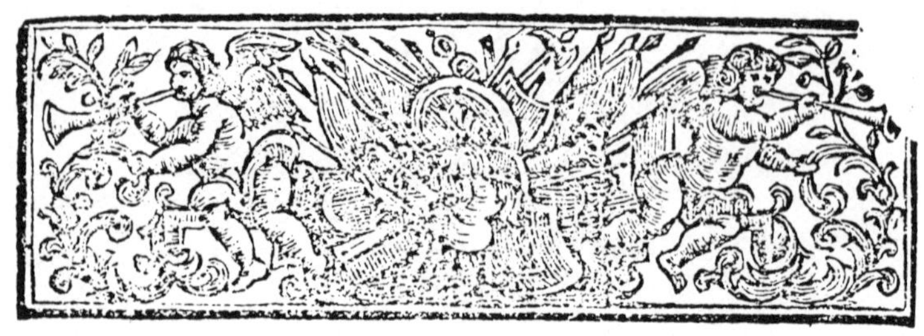

THE DISPENSARY.

CANTO V.

WHEN the ſtill Night, with peaceful Poppies crown'd,
Had ſpread her ſhady Pinions o'er the Ground;
And ſlumb'ring Chiefs of painted Triumphs dream,
While Groves and Streams are the ſoft Virgin's Theme;
The Surges gently daſh againſt the Shoar,
Flocks quit the Plains, and Gally-Slaves the Oar;
Sleep ſhakes its downy Wings o'er mortal Eyes,
Mirmillo is the only Wretch it flies:
He finds no Reſpite from his anxious Grief;
Then ſeeks, from this Soliloquy, Relief.

Long have I reign'd unrival'd in the Town,
Oppreſs'd with Fees and deafen'd with Renown.

None

None e'er cou'd die with due Solemnity,
Unleſs his Paſs-port firſt was ſign'd by Me.
My arbitrary Bounty's undeny'd ;
I give Reverſions, and for Heirs provide.
None cou'd the tedious Nuptial State Support ;
But I, to make it eaſie, make it ſhort.
I ſet the diſcontented Matrons free,
And ranſom Husbands from Captivity.
Shall one of ſuch Importance then engage
In noiſie Riot, and in civil Rage ?
No : I'll endeavour ſtrait a Peace, and ſo
Preſerve my Character, and Perſon too.

But *Diſcord*, that ſtill haunts with hideous Mien
Thoſe dire Abodes where *Hymen* once has been,
O'er-heard *Mirmillo*'s Anguiſh ; then begun
In peeviſh Accents to expreſs her own.

Have I ſo often baniſh'd lazy *Peace*
From her dark Solitude, and lov'd Receſs ?
Have I made *S----th* and *Sh----ck* diſagree,
And puzzle Truth with learn'd Obſcurity ?
And does my faithful *F---ſon* profeſs
His Ardour ſtill for Animoſities ?
Have I, *Britannia*'s Safety to inſure,
Expos'd her naked, to be moſt ſecure ?
Have I made Parties oppoſite, unite,
In monſtrous Leagues of amicable Spight,
To curſe their Country, whilſt the common Cry
Is *Freedom*, but their Aim, the *Miniſtry* ?
And ſhall a Daſtard's Cowardiſe prevent
The War, ſo long I've labour'd to foment ?

No, 'tis resolv'd, he either shall comply,
Or I'll renounce my wan Divinity.

With that, the *Hag* approach'd *Mirmillo*'s Bed,
And taking *Querpo*'s meager Shape, She said;

At Noon of Night I hasten, to dispel
Those Tumults in your pensive Bosom dwell.
I dreamt but now I heard your heaving Sighs,
Nay, saw the Tears debating in your Eyes.
O that 'twere but a Dream! But Threats I find
Low'r in your Looks, and rankle in your Mind.
Speak, whence it is this late Disorder flows,
That shakes your Soul, and troubles your Repose.
Mistakes in Practice scarce cou'd give you Pain,
Too well you know the Dead will ne'er complain.

What Looks discover said the Homicide,
Wou'd be a fruitless Industry to hide.
My Safety first I must consult, and then
I'll serve our suff'ring Party with my Pen.

All shou'd, reply'd the Hag, their Talent learn;
The most attempting oft the least discern.
Let *P-------* speak, and *V-----k* write,
Soft *Acon* court, and rough *Cæcinna* fight:
Such must succeed; but when th' Enervate aim
Beyond their Force, they still contend for Shame.
Had *C-----* printed nothing of his own,
He had not been the *S----fold* o' the Town.
Asses and Owls, unseen their Kind betray,
If these attempt to Hoot, or those to Bray.

Had

Had *W-----* never aim'd in Verse to please,
We had not rank'd him with our *Ogilbys*.
Still Censures will on dull Pretenders fall,
A *Codrus* shou'd expect a *Juvenal*.
Ill Lines, but like ill Paintings, are allow'd,
To set off, and to recommend the good.
So *Diamonds* take a Lustre from their Foyle;
And to a *B----ly* 'tis, we owe a *B----le*.

Consider well the Talent you possess,
To strive to make it more would make it less;
And recollect what Gratitude is due,
To those whose Party you abandon now.
To them you owe your odd Magnificence,
But to your Stars your Magazine of Sense.
Haspt in a Tombril, aukward have you shin'd
With one fat Slave before, and none behind,
Then haste and join your true intrepid Friends,
Success on Vigour and Dispatch attends.

Lab'ring in Doubts *Mirmillo* stood, then said,
'Tis hard to undertake, if Gain disswade;
What Fool for noisie Feuds large Fees wou'd leave?
Ten Harvests more, wou'd all I wish forgive.

True Man, reply'd the Elf; by Choice diseas'd,
Ever contriving Pain, and never pleas'd.
A present Good they slight, an absent chuse,
And what they have, for what they have not, lose.
False Prospects all their true Delights destroy,
Resolv'd to want, yet lab'ring to enjoy.

In reſtleſs Hurries thoughtleſly they live,
At Subſtance oft unmov'd, for Shadows grieve.
Children at Toys, as Men at Titles aim;
And in effect both covet but the ſame.
This *Philip*'s Son prov'd in revolving Years;
And firſt for Rattles, then for Worlds ſhed Tears.

The Fury ſpoke, then in a Moment fir'd
The Heroe's Breaſt with Tempeſts, and retir'd.

In boding Dreams *Mirmillo* ſpent the Night,
And frightful Phantoms danc'd before his Sight,
Till the pale *Pleiads* clos'd their Eyes of Light.
At length gay Morn glows in the Eaſtern Skies,
The Larks in Raptures thro' the *Æther* riſe,
The Azure Miſts ſcud o'er the dewy Lawns,
The *Chaunter* at his early Matins yawns,
The *Amaranth* opes its Leaves, the *Lys* its Bells,
And *Progne* her Complaint of *Tereus* tells.

As bold *Mirmillo* the gray Dawn deſcries,
Arm'd *Cap-a-pe*, where Honour calls, he flies,
And finds the Legions planted at their Poſt;
Where mighty *Querpo* fill'd the Eye the moſt.
His Arms were made, if we may credit Fame,
By * *Mulciber* the Mayor of *Bromingham*,
Of temper'd *Stibium* the bright Shield was caſt,
† And yet the Work the Metal far ſurpaſs'd.

* *See the Alluſion* Hom. Il. *B.* 18. Virg. Æn. *B.* 8.
† *See* Ov. Met. *B.* 2.

A Foliage of the Vulnerary Leaves,
Grav'd round the Brim, the wond'ring Sight deceives.
Around the Center Fate's bright Trophies lay,
Probes, Saws, Incision Knives, and Tools to flay.
Emboft upon the Field, a Battel ftood
Of *Leeches* fpouting *Hemorrhoidal* Blood.
The Artift too expref's'd the folemn State
Of grave *Phyficians* at a Confult met;
About each Symptom how they difagree,
But how unanimous in cafe of Fee.
Whilft each *Affaffion* his learn'd Collegue tires
With learn'd Impertinence, the Sick expires.

Beneath this blazing Orb bright *Querpo* fhone,
Himfelf an *Atlas*, and his Shield a Moon.
A Peftle for his Truncheon led the Van,
And his high Helmet was a Clofe-ftool Pan.
His Creft an † *Ibis*, brandifhing her Beak,
And winding in loofe Folds her fpiral Neck.
This, when the Young * *Querpoides* beheld,
His Face in Nurfe's Breaft the Boy conceal'd;
Then peept, and with th' effulgent Helm wou'd play,
And as the Monfter gap'd wou'd fhrink away.
Thus fometimes Joy prevail'd, and fometimes Fear;
And Tears and Smiles alternate Paffions were.

As *Querpo* tow'ring ftood in Martial Might,
Pacifick *Carus* fparkled on the Right.

† *This Bird, according to the Ancients, gives it felf a Clyfter with its Beak.*

* *Alluding to* Aftyanax. *See* Hom. II.

An

An * *Oran Outang* o'er his Shoulders hung,
His plume confeſs'd the Capon whence it ſprung.
His motly Mail ſcarce cou'd the Heroe bear,
Haranguing thus the Tribunes of the War.

Fam'd Chiefs,
For preſent Triumphs born, deſign'd for more,
Your Virtue I admire, your Valour more,
If Battel be reſolv'd, you'll find this Hand
Can deal out Deſtiny, and Fate command.
Our Foes in Throngs ſhall hide the Crimſon Plain,
And their *Apollo* interpoſe in vain.
Tho' Gods themſelves engage, a † *Diamed*
With eaſe cou'd ſhow a *Deity* can bleed.

But War's rough Trade ſhou'd be by Fools profeſt,
The trueſt Rubbiſh fills the Trench the beſt.
Let Quinſies throttle, and the Quartan ſhake,
Or Dropſies drown, and Gout and Cholicks rack;
Let Sword and Peſtilence lay waſte, whilſt we
Wage bloodleſs Wars, and fight in Theory.
Who wants not Merit needs not arm for Fame;
The Dead I raiſe my Chivalry proclaim,
Diſeaſes baffled, and loſt Health reſtor'd,
In Fame's bright Liſt my Victories record.
More Lives from me their Preſervation own,
Than Lovers loſe if Fair *Cornelia* frown.

Your Cures, ſhrill *Querpo* cry'd aloud you tell,
But wiſely your Miſcarriages conceal.

* *The Skin of a diſected Baboon call'd ſo.*

† *See* Hom. Il. *B.* 5.

Zeno

Zeno, a Prieſt, in *Samothrace* of old,
Thus reaſon'd with *Philopidas* the bold;
Immortal Gods you own, but think 'em blind
To what concerns the State of human kind.
Either they hear not, or regard not Pray'r,
That argues want of Pow'r, and this of Care.
Allow that Wiſdom infinite muſt know:
Pow'r infinite muſt act. *I grant it ſo.*
Haſte ſtrait to *Neptune's* Fane, ſurvey with Zeal
The Walls. *What then?* reply'd the Infidel.
Obſerve thoſe numerous Throngs in Effigy,
The Gods have ſav'd from the devouring Sea.
'Tis true, their Pictures that eſcap'd you keep,
But where are theirs that periſh'd in the deep?

Vaunt now no more the Triumph of your Skill,
But, tho' unfee'd, exert your Arm and kill.
Our Scouts have learn'd the poſture of the Foe;
In War, Surprizes ſureſt Conduct ſhow.

But Fame, that neither good nor bad conceals,
That *P- - - -k's* Worth, and *O- - - -*'s Valour tells;
How Truth in *B- - - -*, how in *C- - - -ſh* reigns
Varro's Magnificence with *Maro's* Strains;
But how at Church and Bar all gape and ſtretch
If *W- - - - -* plead, or *S- - - -* or *O- - -ly* preach;
On nimble Wings to *Warwick-Lane* repairs,
And what the Enemy intends, declares.
Confuſion in each Countenance appear'd,
A Council's call'd, and *Stentor* firſt was heard;
His lab'ring Lungs the throng'd *Prætorium* rent,
Addreſſing thus the paſſive Preſident.

Machaon,

Machaon, whoſe Experience we adore,
Great as your matchleſs Merit, is your Pow'r.
At your Approach, the baffled Tyrant *Death*
Breaks his keen Shafts, and grind his claſhing Teeth.
To you we leave the Conduct of the Day;
What you command your Vaſſals muſt obey.
If this dread Enterprize you wou'd decline,
We'll ſend to treat, and ſtifle the Deſign.
But if my Arguments had Force, we'd try
To humble our audacious Foes, or die,
Our Spight, they'll find, to their Advantage leans,
The End is good, no matter for the means.
So modern *Caſuiſts* their Talents try,
Uprightly for the ſake of Truth to lye.

He had not finiſh'd, 'till th' Out-guards deſcry'd
Bright Columns move in formidable Pride.
The paſſing Pomp ſo dazzled from afar,
It ſeem'd a Triumph, rather than a War.
Tho' wide the Front, tho' groſs the *Phalanx* grew,
It look'd leſs dreadful, as it nearer drew.

The adverſe Hoſt for Action ſtraight prepare;
All eager to unveil the Face of War.
Their Chiefs lace on their Helms, and take the Field,
And to their truſty Squires reſign their Shield:
To paint each Knight, their Ardour and Alarms,
Wou'd ask the Muſe that ſung the Frogs in Arms.

And now the Signal ſummons to the Fray;
Mock Falchions flaſh, and Paltry Enſigns Play.

Their

Their Patron God his ſilver Bow-ſtring twangs;
Tough Harneſs ruſtles, and bold Armour clangs.
The piercing *Cauſticks* ply their ſpightful Pow'r;
Emeticks ranch, and keen *Catharticks* ſcour.
The deadly Drugs in double Doſes fly;
And Peſtles peal a martial Symphony.

Now from their levell'd *Syringes* they pour
The liquid Volly of a Miſſive Show'r.
Not Storms of Sleet, which o'er the *Baltick* drive.
Puſh'd on by *Northern* Guſts, ſuch Horror give.
Like Spouts in *Southern* Seas the Deluge broke,
And Numbers ſunk beneath th' impetuous Stroke.

So when *Leviathans* diſpute the Reign
And uncontroul'd Dominion of the Main
From the rent Rocks whole *Coral* Groves are torn,
And Iſles of *Sea-weed* on the Waves are born.
Such watry Stores from their ſpread Noſtrils fly.
'Tis doubtful which is Sea, and which is Sky.

And now the ſtagg'ring *Braves*, led by Deſpair.
Advance, and to return the Charge, prepare.
Each ſeizes for his Shield a ſpacious *Scale*,
And the *Braſs Weights* fly thick as Show'rs of Hail,
Whole Heaps of Warriors welter on the Ground,
With Gally-pots, and broken Phials crown'd
Whilſt empty Jars the dire Defeat reſound.

Thus when ſome Storm its Cryſtal Quarry rends,
And *Jove* in rattling Show'rs of *Ice* deſcends;

Mount *Athos* ſhakes, the Forreſts on his Brow,
Whilſt down his wounded Sides freſh Torrents flow,
And Leaves and Limbs of Trees o'erſpread the Vale
(below.

But now, all Order loſt, promiſcuous Blows
Confus'dly fall; perplex'd the Battle grows.
From *Stertor's* Arm a maſſy Opiat flyes,
And ſtrait a deadly Sleep clos'd *Carus'* Eyes.
At *Colon* great *Sertorious* Buckthorn flung,
Who with fierce Gripes, like thoſe of Death, was ſtung.
But with a dauntleſs and diſdainful Mien
Hurl'd back Steel Pills, and hit him on the Spleen.
Chiron attack'd *Talthibius* with ſuch Might,
One Paſs had paunch'd the huge hydropick Knight,
Who ſtrait retreated to evade the Wound,
But in a Flood of *Apozem* was drown'd.
This *Pſylas* ſaw, and to the Victor ſaid,
Thou ſhalt not long ſurvive th' unwieldy Dead.
Thy Fate ſhall follow; to confirm it, ſwore
By th'Image of *Priapus*, which he bore:
And rais'd an * *Eagle-ſtone*, invoking loud
On *Cynthia*, leaning o'er a Silver Cloud.

Great Queen of Night, and Empreſs of the Seas,
If faithful to thy Midnight Myſteries,
If ſtill obſervant of my early Vows,
Theſe Hands have eas'd the mourning Matron's Throws,
Direct this rais'd avenging Arm aright,
So may loud Cymbals aid thy lab'ring Light.
He ſaid, and let the pond'rous Fragment fly
At *Chiron*, but learn'd *Hermes* put it by.

* *See* Plin.

Tho'

Tho' the haranguing God ſurvey'd the War,
That Day the Muſes Sons were not his Care.
Two Friends, Adepts, the *Triſmegiſts* by Name,
Alike their Features, and alike their Flame.
As ſimpling ne'er fair *Tweed* each ſung by turn,
The liſt'ning River wou'd neglect his Urn.
Thoſe Lives they fail'd to reſcue by their Skill,
Their * Muſe cou'd make immortal with her Quill.
But learn'd Enquiries after Nature's State
Diſſolv'd the League, and kindled a Debate.
The one for lofty Labours fruitful known,
Fill'd Magazines with Volumes of his own.
At his once-favour'd Friend a Tome he threw
That from his birth had ſlept unſeen 'till now.
Stunn'd with a blow the batter'd Bard retir'd
Sunk down, and in a *Simile* expir'd.

And now the Cohorts ſhake, the Legions ply,
The yielding Flanks confeſs the Victory.
Stentor undaunted ſtill, with noble Rage
Sprung thro' the Battel, *Querpo* to engage.
Fierce was the Onſet, the Diſpute was great.
Both cou'd not vanquiſh, Neither wou'd retreat;
Each Combatant his Adverſary mauls,
With batter'd *Bed-pans*, and ſtarv'd *Urinals*.
On *Stentor's* Creſt the uſeful Chryſtal breaks,
And Tears of *Amber* gutter'd down his Cheeks.
But whilſt the Champion, as late Rumours tell,
Deſign'd a ſure deciſive Stroke, he fell:
And as the Victor hov'ring o'er him ſtood,
With Arms extended, thus the *Suppliant* ſu'd,

* *See* Taſs.

When

When Honour's loſt, 'tis a relief to die:
Death's but a ſure Retreat from infamy.
But to the loſt, if Pity might be ſhown,
Reflect on young, *Querpoides* thy Son;
Then pity mine, for ſuch an Infant-Grace
Smiles in his Eyes, and flatters in his Face.
If he was near, Compaſſion he'd create,
Or elſe lament his wretched Parent's Fate.
Thine is the Glory, and the Field is thine;
To thee the lov'd * *Diſpens'ry* I reſign.

At this the *Victors* own ſuch Ecſtas,
As *Memphian* Prieſts if their *Oſiris* ſneeze:
Or Champions with Olympick Clangour fir'd;
Or ſimpring Prudes with ſprightly *Nantz* inſpir'd;
Or Sultans rais'd from Dungeons to a Crown;
Or faſting Zealots when the Sermon's done.

A While the Chief the deadly Stroak declin'd,
And found Compaſſion pleading in his Mind.
But whilſt he view'd with Pity the diſtreſs'd,
He ſpy'd † *Signetur* writ upon his Breaſt
Then tow'rds the Skies he toſs'd his threatning Head.
And fir'd with more than mortal Fury, ſaid,

Sooner than I'll from vow'd Revenge deſiſt,
His *Holineſs* ſhall turn a *Quietiſt*,
Janſenius and the *Jeſuits* agree,
The Inquiſition wink at Hereſie,

* *See the Alluſion*, Virg. Æn.

† *Thoſe Members of the Colledge that obſerve a late Statute, are call'd by the Apothecaries* Signetur Men.

Warm

Warm Convocations own the Church ſecure,
And more conſult her Doctrine than her Pow'r.

With that he drew a Lancet in his Rage,
To puncture the ſtill ſupplicating Sage.
But while his Thoughts that fatal ſtroke decree,
Apollo interpos'd in form of Fee.
The *Chief* great *Pæan's* golden Treſſes knew,
He own'd the God, and his rais'd Arm withdrew.

Thus often at the *Temple-Stairs* we've ſeen
Two Tritons of a rough Athletick Mien,
Sourly diſpute ſome Quarrel of the Flood,
With Knuckles bruis'd, and Face beſmear'd in Blood.
But at the firſt Appearance of a Fare,
Both quit the Fray, and to their Oars repair.

The Heroe ſo his Enterprize recalls,
His Fiſt unclinches, and the Weapon falls.

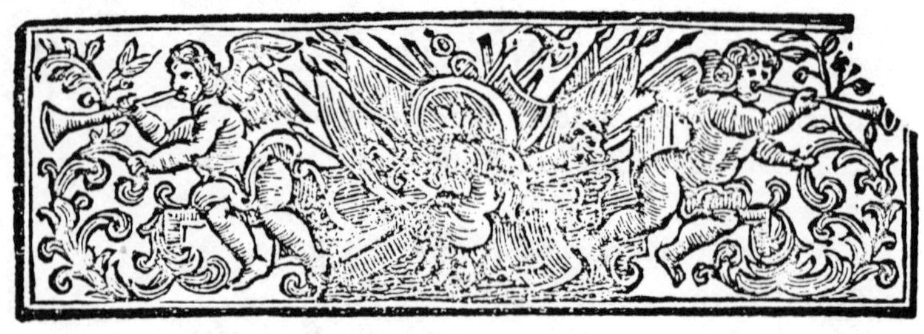

THE DISPENSARY.

CANTO VI.

WHile the shrill Clangour of the Battle rings,
Auspicious *Health* appear'd on *Zephir*'s Wings;
She seem'd a Cherub most divinely bright.
More soft than Air, more gay than Morning Light,
A Charm she takes from each excelling Fair,
And borrows *C----le*'s Shape, and G----*ton*'s Air.
Her Eyes like R----*agh*'s their Beams dispense,
With *Ch---ill*'s Bloom, and *B---kley*'s Innocence;
On *Iris* thus the differing * Beams bestow
The Die, that paints the Wonders of her Bow;
From the fair Nymph a vocal Musick falls,
As to *Machaon* thus the Goddess calls.

Enough th' Atchievement of your Arms you've shown,
You seek a Triumph you shou'd blush to own.

* *See* Newt. *of Col*.

Haste

Haste to th' *Elysian* Fields, those bless'd Aboads,
Where Harvy sits among the Demi-Gods.
Consult the sacred Sage, soon He'll disclose
The Method that most mollify these Woes.
Let *Celsus* for that Enterprize prepare,
His Conduct to the Shades shall be my Care.

Aghast the Heroes stood dissolv'd in Fear,
A Form so Heav'nly bright They cou'd not bear;
Celsus alone unmov'd, the Sight beheld,
The rest in pale Confusion left the Field.

So when the Pigmies, marshall'd on the Plains,
Wage puny War against th'invading Cranes;
The Poppets to their Bodkin Spears repair,
And scatter'd Feathers flutter in the Air;
But when the bold imperial Bird of *Jove*
Stoops on his sounding Pinions from above,
Among the Brakes the Fairy Nation crowds,
And the *Strimonian* squadron seeks the Clouds.

And now the Delegate prepares to go
And view the Wonders of the Realms below;
Then takes *Amomum* for the Golden Bough.
Thrice did the Goddess with her Sacred Wand
The Pavement strike; and strait at her Command
The willing Surface opens, and descries
A deep Descent that leads to nether Skies.
* *Hygeia* to the silent Region tends;
And with his Heav'nly Guide the *Charge* descends.

* *Health, celebrated by the Ancients as a Goddess.*

Thus

Thus *Numa* when to hallow'd Caves retir'd,
Was by * *Ægeria* guarded and inſpir'd.

Within the Chambers of the Globe they ſpy
The Beds where ſleeping Vegetables lye,
'Till the glad Summons of a genial Ray
Unbinds the Glebe, and calls them out to Day.
Hence *Pancies* trick themſelves in various Hew,
And hence *Junquils* derive their fragrant Dew;
Hence the *Carnation* and the baſhful *Roſe*
Their Virgin Bluſhes to the Morn diſcloſe.
Hence the chaſt *Lilly* riſes to the Light,
Unveils her ſnowy Breaſts, and charms the Sight,
Hence Arbours are with twining Greens array'd.
T'oblige complaining Lovers with their Shade,
And hence on *Daphne's* Laurell'd Forehead grow
Immortal Wreaths for *Phœbus* and *Naſſau*.

The Inſects here their lingring Trance ſurvive:
Benum'd they ſeem, and doubtful if alive.
From Winter's Fury hither they repair,
And ſtay for milder Skies and ſofter Air,
Down to theſe Cells obſcener Reptils creep,
Where hateful *Nutes* and painted *Lizzards* ſleep.
Where ſhiv'ring *Snakes* the Summer Solrice wait;
Unfurl their painted Folds, and ſlide in State.
Here their new Form the numb'd † *Eruca* hide,
Their num'rous Feet in ſlender Bandage ty'd:
Soon as the kindling Year begins to riſe,
This upſtart Race their native clod deſpiſe
And proud of painted Wings attempt the Skies.

* *See Ov. Met. B.* 15.

† *See* Gordort *of Caterpillars and Butterflies.*

Now

Now these profounder Regions They explore,
Where Metals ripen in vast Cakes of Oar.
Here, sullen to the sight, at large is spread
The dull unwieldy Mass of lumpish Lead.
There, glimm'ring in their dawning Beds, are seen
The more aspiring Seeds of sprightly Tin.
The * Copper sparkles next in rudy Streaks;
And in the gloom betrays its glowing Cheeks.
The Silver then with bright and burnish'd Grace,
Youth and a blooming Lustre in its Face,
To th' Arms of those more yielding Metals flies,
And in the Folds of their Embraces lyes.
So close they cling, so stubbornly retire;
Their Love's more violent than the Chymist's Fire.

Near these the Delegate with wonder spies
Where Floods of living Silver serpentize:
Where richest Metals their bright looks put on,
And Golden Streams through Amber Channels run.
Where Lights gay God descends to ripen Gems,
And lend a Lustre brighter than his Beams.

Here he observes the Subteranean Cells,
Where wanton Nature sports in idle Shells.
Some *Helicoeids*; some *Comical* appear;
These, Miters emulate; those, Turbans are.
Here Marcasites in various Figure wait.
To ripen to a true Metallick State:
Till Drops that from impending Rocks descend
Their Substance petrifie, and Progress End.
Nigh, livid Seas of kindled Sulphur flow;
And, whilst enrag'd, their fiery Surges glow:

* *See* Yald. *on Mines.*

Convul-

Convulſions in the lab'ring Mountains riſe,
And hurl their melted Vitals to the Skies.

He views with Horror next the noiſie Cave,
Where with hoarſe Dinns impriſon'd Tempeſts rave;
Where clam'rous Hurricanes attempt their Flight,
Or, whirling in tumultuous Eddies, fight.
The warring Winds unmov'd *Hygeia* heard,
Brav'd their loud Jars, but much for *Celſus* fear'd.
Andromeda, ſo whilſt her Heroe fought,
Shook for his Danger, but her own forgot.

And now the Goddeſs with her Charge deſcends,
Where ſcarce one chearful Glimpſe their Steps befriends.
Here his forſaken Seat old *Chaos* keeps;
And undiſturb'd by Form in Silence ſleeps.
A griſly Wight, and hideous to the Eye;
An aukward Lump of ſhapeleſs Anarchy.
With ſordid Age his Features are defac'd;
His Lands unpeopled, and his Countries waſte.
To theſe dark Realms much learned Lumber creeps,
There copious *M*- - - -ſafe in Silence ſleeps.
Where Muſhroom Libels in Oblivion lie,
And, ſoon as born, like other Monſters die.
Upon a Couch of *Jett* in theſe Abodes,
Dull *Night*, his melancholly Conſort, nods.
No ways and Means their Cabinet employ;
But their dark Hours they waſte in barren Joy.

Nigh this Receſs, with Terror they ſurvey
Where *Death* maintains his dread tyrannick Sway;
In the cloſe Covert of a Cypreſs Grove,
Where *Goblins* friſk, and airy *Spectres* rove,

Yawns

Yawns a dark Cave, with awful Horror wide,
And there the *Monarch*'s Triumphs are defcry'd.
Confus'd, and wildly huddled to the Eye,
The Beggars Pouch, and Prince's Purple lye.
Dim Lamps with fickly Rays fcarce feem to glow;
Sighs heave in mournful Moans, and Tears o'er-flow.
Reftlefs Anxiety, forlorn Defpair,
And all the faded Family of Care.
Old mouldring Urns, Racks, Daggers and Diftrefs
Make up the frightful Horror o'the Place.

Within its dreadful Jaws thofe Furies wait,
Which execute the harfh Decrees of Fate.
* *Febris* is firft: The *Hag* relentlefs hears
The Virgin's Sighs; and fees the Infant's Tears.
In her parch'd Eye-Balls fiery *Meteors* reign;
And reftlefs Ferments revel in each Vein.

Then † *Hydrops* next appears amongft the Throng;
Bloated, and big, fhe flowly fails along.
But, like a Mifer, in Excefs fhe's poor;
And pines for thirft amidft her wat'ry Store,

Now loathfome ‖ *Lepra*, that offenfive Spright,
With foul Eruptions ftain'd offends the Sight,
Still deaf to Beauty's foft perfuading Pow'r:
Nor can bright *Hebe*'s Charms her Bloom fecure.

Whilft meager ¶ *Pthifis* gives a filent Blow;
Her Strokes are fure; but her Advances flow.
No loud Alarms, nor fierce Affaults are fhown:
She ftarves the *Fortrefs* firft; then takes the *Town*.

* *Feaver.* † *Dropfie.* ‖ *Leprofie.* ¶ *Confumption.*

Behind

Behind ſtood Crouds of much inferior Name,
Too num'rous to repeat, too foul to name;
The Vaſſals of their Monarch's Tyranny:
Who, at his Nod, on fatal Errands fly.

Now *Celſus*, with his glorious Guide, invades
The ſilent Region of the fleeting Shades:
Where Rocks and ruful Deſarts are deſcry'd;
And ſullen *Styx* rolls down his lazy Tide.
Then ſhews the Ferryman the Plant he bore,
And claims his Paſſage to the further Shore.
To whom the *Stygian Pilot* ſmiling, ſaid,
You need no Paſs-port to demand our Aid.
Phyſicians never linger on this Strand:
Old *Charon*'s preſent ſtill at their Command.
Our awful Monarch and his Conſort owe
To them the peopling of their Realms below.
Then in his ſwarthy Hand he graſp'd his Oar,
Receiv'd his Gueſts aboard, and ſhov'd from Shoar.

Now, as the Goddeſs and her *Charge* prepare
To breath the Sweets of ſoft *Elyſian* Air,
Upon the Left thy ſpy a penſive * Shade,
Who on his bended Arm had rais'd his Head:
Pale Grief ſat heavy on his mournful Look:
To whom not unconcern'd, thus *Celſus* ſpoke:

Tell me, thou much afflicted Shade, why Sighs
Burſt from your Breaſt, and Torrents from your Eyes:
And who thoſe mangled *Manes* are, which ſhow
A ſullen Satisfaction at your Woe?

* *See the Alluſion.* Virg. Æn. B. 6.

Sinceo

Since, said the Ghost, with Pity you'll attend,
Know, I'm *Guiacum* once your firmest Friend.
And on this barren Beach in Discontent
Am doom'd to stay, 'till th'angry Pow'rs relent.
Those *Spectres* seam'd with Scars that threaten there,
The Victims of my late ill Conduct are.
They vex with endless Clamours my Repose:
This wants his Palate; That demands his Nose:
And here they execute stern *Pluto*'s Will,
And ply me ever'y Moment with a Pill.

Then *Celsus* thus, O much-lamented State,
How rigid is the Sentence you relate?
Methinks I recollect your former Air,
But ah, how much you're chang'd from what you were.
Insipid as your late *Ptisans* you lye,
That once were sprightlier far than *Mercury*.
At the sad Tale you tell, the Poppies weep,
And mourn their vegetable Souls asleep.
The unctuous *Larix*, and the healing *Pine*
Lament your Fate in Tears of Turpentine.
But still the Off-spring of your Brain shall prove
The Grocer's Care, and brave the Rage of *Jove*.
When Bonfires blaze, your vagrant Works shall rise
In Rockets, 'till they reach the Wond'ring Skies.

If Mortals e'er the *Stygian* Pow'rs cou'd bend,
Entreaties to their awful Seats I'd send.
But since no human Arts the Fates dissuade;
Direct me how to find bless'd *Harvy*'s Shade.
In vain th' unhappy Ghost still urg'd his Stay;
Then rising from the Ground, he shew'd the Way.

Nigh the dull Shoar a shapeless Mountain stood,
That with a dreadful Frown survey'd the Flood.
Its fearful Brow no lively Greens put on,
No frisking Goats bound o'er the ridgy Stone.
To gain the Summit the bright Goddess try'd,
And *Celsus* follow'd, by degrees, his Guide.

Th' Ascent thus conquer'd, now they towre on high,
And taste th' Indulgence of a milder Sky.
Loose *Breezes* on their airy Pinions play,
Soft Infant Blossoms their chast Odours pay;
And Roses blush their fragrant Lives away.
Cool Streams thro' flow'ry Meadows gently glide;
And as they pass, their painted Banks they chide.
These blissful Plains no Blights, nor Mildews fear,
The Flow'rs ne'er fade, and Shrubs are Myrtles here.
The Morn awakes the Tulip from her Bed;
E'er Noon in painted Pride she decks her Head:
Roab'd in rich Dye she triumphs on the Green,
And ev'ry Flow'r does Homage to their Queen.
So when bright *Venus* rises from the Flood,
Around in Throngs the wond'ring *Nereids* crowd;
The *Tritons* gaze, and tune each vocal Shell,
And ev'ry Grace unsung, the Waves conceal.

The *Delegate* observes, with wond'ring Eyes,
Ambrosial Dews descend, and Incense rise.
Then hastens onward to the pensive Grove,
The silent * *Mansion* of disastrous Love.
Here Jealousie with Jaundice Looks appears,
And broken Slumbers, and fantastick Fears.

* *See* Virg. Æn. B. 6.

The

The widow'd Turtle hangs her moulting Wings,
And to the Woods in mournful Murmurs ſings.
No Winds but Sighs there are, no Floods but Tears.
Each conſcious Tree a Tragick Signal bears.
Their wounded Bark records ſome broken Vow,
And Willow Garlands hang on ev'ry Bough.

Olivia here in Solitude he found,
Her down-caſt Eyes fix'd on the ſilent Ground:
Her Dreſs neglected, and unbound her Hair,
She ſeem'd the dying Image of Deſpair.
How lately did this celebrated *Thing*
Blaze in the Box, and ſparkle in the Ring.
'Till the Green-ſickneſs and Love's force betray'd
To Death's remorſeleſs Arms, th' unhappy Maid.

All o'er confus'd the guilty Lover ſtood,
The Light forſook his Eyes, his Cheeks the Blood;
An Icy Horrour ſhiver'd in his Look,
As to the cold-complexion'd Nymph He ſpoke:

Tell me, dear Shade, from whence ſuch anxious Care,
Your Looks diſorder'd, and your Boſom bare?
Why thus you languiſh like a drooping Flow'r.
Cruſh'd by the weight of ſome relentleſs Show'r?
Your languid Looks, your late ill Conduct tell;
O that inſtead of Traſh you'd taken Steel!

Stabb'd with th' unkind Reproach, the Conſcious Maid
Thus to her late inſulting Lover ſaid;
When Ladies liſten not to looſe Deſire
You ſtile our Modeſty, our want of Fire.

Smile or forbid, Encourage or Reprove,
You ſtill find Reaſons to believe we love:
Vainly you think a liking we betray,
And never mean the peeviſh Things we ſay.
Few are the Fair Ones of *Rufilla's* make,
Unask'd ſhe grants, uninjur'd ſhe'll forſake:
But ſev'ral *Cælia's*, ſev'ral Ages boaſt,
That like, where Reaſon recommends the moſt.
Where heav'nly Truth and Tenderneſs conſpire,
Chaſt Paſſion may Perſwade us to deſire.

Your Sex, he cry'd, as Cuſtom bids, behaves;
In Forms the Tyrant tyes ſuch haughty Slaves.
To do nice Conduct Right, you Nature wrong;
Impulſes are but weak, where Reaſon's ſtrong.
Some want the Courage, but how Few the Flame!
They like the Thing, that ſtartle at the Name.
The lonely *Phænix*, tho' profeſs'd a Nun,
Warms into Love, and kindles at the Sun.
Thoſe Tales of Spicy Urns and fragrant Fires,
Are but the Emblems of her ſcorch'd Deſires.

Then as he ſtrove to claſp the fleeting *Fair*,
His empty Arms confeſs'd th' impaſſive Air.
From his embrace th' unbody'd Spectre flies,
And as ſhe mov'd, ſhe chid him with her Eyes.

They haſten now to that delightful Plain,
Where the glad *Manes* of the bleſs'd remain:
Where *Harvey* gathers Simples, to beſtow
Immortal Youth on Heroe's Shades below.
Soon as the bright *Hygeia* was in view,
The Venerable Sage her Preſence knew;
Thus he- - -

Hail,

Hail, blooming Goddess! Thou propitious Pow'r,
Whose Blessings Mortals more than Life implore.
With so much Lustre your bright Looks endear,
That Cottages are Courts where those appear.
Mankind, as you vouchsafe to smile or frown,
Finds ease in Chains, or anguish in a Crown.

With just Resentments and Contempt you see
The foul Dissentions of the *Faculty*;
How your sad sick'ning Art now hangs her Head,
And once a Science, is become a Trade.
Her Sons ne'er rifle her Mysterious Store,
But study Nature less, and Lucre more.
Not so when *Rome* to th' *Epidaurian* rais'd
A * Temple, where devoted Incence blaz'd.
Oft Father *Tyber* views the lofty Fire,
As the learn'd Son is worship'd like the Sire;
The Sage with *Romulus* like Honours claim;
The Gift of Life and Laws were then the same,

I show'd of old, how vital Currents glide.
And the *Meanders* of their refluent Tide.
Then, *Willis*, why spontaneous Actions here,
And whence involuntary Motions there,
And how the Spirits by Mechanick Laws,
In wild Careers, tumultuous Riots Cause.
Nor wou'd our *Wharton*, *Bates*, and *Glisson* lye
In the Abyss of blind Obscurity.
But now such wond'rous Searches are forborn,
And *Pæans* Art is by Divisions torn.

* *A Temple built at* Rome, *in the Island of* Tyber, *to* Æsculapius *Son of* Apollo.

Then let your *Charge* attend, and I'll explain
How her lost Health your Science may regain.

Haste, and the matchless *Atticus* Addrefs,
From Heav'n and great *Nassau* he has the Mace.
Th' oppress'd to his *Asylum* still repair;
Arts he supports, and Learning is his Care.
He softens the harsh Rigour of the Laws,
Blunts their keen Edge, and grinds their Harpy Claws;
And graciously he casts a pitying Eye
On the sad State of virtuous poverty.
Whene'er he speaks, Heav'ns! how the list'ning Throng
Dwells on the melting Musick of his Tongue.
His Arguments are Emblems of his Mein,
Mild, but not faint; and forcing, tho' serene;
And when the Pow'r of Eloquence he'd try,
Here, Light'ning strikes you; there, soft breezes sigh.

To him you must your sickly State refer,
Your Charter claims him as your Visiter.
Your Wounds he'll close, and sov'reignly restore
Your Science to the height it had before.

Then *Nassau*'s Health shall be your glorious Aim,
His Life should be as lasting as his Fame.
Some Princes claims from devastions spring,
He condescends in Pity to be King:
And when, amidst his *Olives* plac'd, he stands,
And governs more by Candour than Commmands:
Ev'n then not less a Heroe he appears,
Than when his *Laurel* Diadem he wears.

Wou'd

Wou'd *Phœbus*, or his *G- - - -le*, but inspire
Their sacred Veh'mence of Poetick Fire;
To celebrate in Song that God-like Pow'r,
Which did the lab'ring Universe restore:
Fair *Albion's* Cliffs wou'd Eccho to the Strain,
And praise the Arm that conquer'd, to regain
The Earth's repose, and Empire o'er the Main.

Still may th' immortal Man his Cares repeat,
To make his blessings endless as they're great:
Whilst *Malice* and *Ingratitude* confess
They've strove for Ruin long without success.
When late, *Jove's* * Eagle from the Pyle shall rise
To bear the Victor to the Boundless Skies,
Awhile the God puts off Paternal Care,
Neglects the Earth, to give the Heav'ns a Star.
Near thee, † *Alcides*, shall the Heroe shine;
His Rays resembling, as his Labours, thine.

Had some fam'd *Patriot*, of the *Latin* Blood,
Like *Julius* Great, and like *Octavius* Good,
But thus preserv'd the *Latian* Liberties,
Aspiring Columns soon had reach'd the Skies:
Loud *Io's* the proud Capitol had shook,
And all the Statues of the Gods had spoke.

No more the Sage his Raptures cou'd pursue:
He paus'd; and *Celsus* with his Guide withdrew.

* *Read the Ceremony of the Apothesis.*

† Hercules, *a Constellation near* Ariadne's *Crown.*

FINIS.

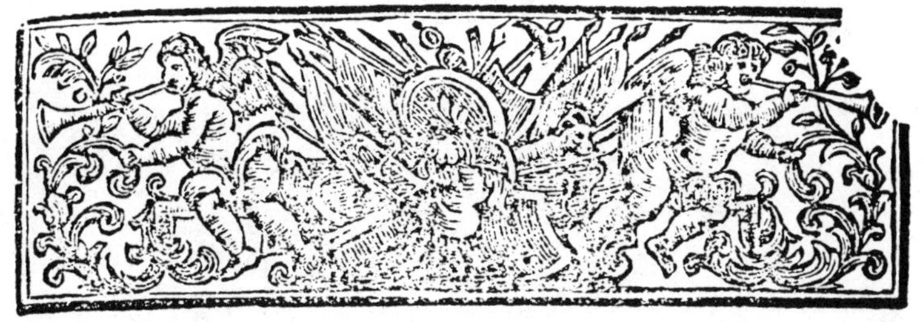

A

Compleat KEY

TO THE

DISPENSARY.

In the Firſt Copy of VERSES. To Dr. *GARTH* upon the *Diſpenſary*.

Lin. 2. LIKE * M----gue's *could a juſt Piece ſuſtain.*
* Charles Montague *Lord* Halifax.

Lin. 15. *When* † S-----rs *Charming Eloquence.*
† The Lord *Somers*, formerly Lord Chancellor.

Lin. 20. *What* ‖ D----s *can't condemn nor* ¶ D---n *mend.*
‖ *Dennis*, a ſower, ſupercillious and ill-natur'd Critick and Poetaſter.
¶ *Dryden*, a famous Poet.

In

In the Second Copy of VERSES, written by the late Colonel *Codrington*, Governor of the *Leeward Islands.*

Lin. 13. THE *Nymph has* 1 G----n's 2 C---l's 3 C--l's *Charms.*

1 The Dutchess of *Grafton.*

2 *Cecil's*, the late Countess of *Salisbury.*

3 The Lady-----*Churchil*, one of the Duke of *Marlborough's* Daughters.

Lin. 22. Lucretius, Horace, 1 S----d, 2 M----ue,

1 *Sheffield*, the Duke of *Buckinghnm* and *Normanby.*

2 *Montague*, Lord *Halifax.*

Lin. 27. *Facetious* 1 M---- *and the City*, 2 B---

1 *Mirmil*, Dr. *Gibbons.*

2 The *City Bard*, Sir *Richard Blackmore.*

Lin 36. *H----s*, Dr. *Hans.*

Lin. 37. R----*e*, Dr. *Ratcliffe.*

Lin. 39. *M----l's*, i. e. *Mirmil's*, Dr. *Gibbons.*

Lin. 42. *W---h*, the late *William Walsh*, Esq;

Lin. 43. To 1 *S---s* and to *D---t* too submit,

1 The Lord *Somers*.

2 The late Earl of *Dorset.*

CANTO I.

Pag. Ver.

2 2. GReat *Naſſau*, the late King *William*, of Glorious and Immortal Memory.

8. *Why* * S----*rages to ſurvive deſire.*

* *Scarſedale*, the late Lord of that Name.

10. *Whence Tropes to* 1 F----, *or Impudence to* 2 S----

1 *Finch*, the preſent Lord *Guernſey*.

2 *Sloan*, a late Lawyer, famous in *Weſtminſter-Hall for his Vociferation and Impudence.*

6 16. Urim *was Civil*, &c.

What *fiery Divine* is here meant by *Urim*, is eaſie to gueſs: 'tis but looking over the Liſts of the *Prolocutors*, and of the Prelates that have filled the See of *Rocheſter*, and then conſider which of them the Character of *Urim* fits beſt.

7 16. *NASSAU*, the late King *WILLIAM*.

CANTO II.

Pag. ver.

12 3. A † Herione *ſhall* Albion's *Scepter bear*.

† Queen *Anne*, whoſe Triumphs ſhall ever ſhine in *Britiſh* Annals.

13 1. Colon---Mr. *Lee*, an Apothecary.

7. Horoſcope, *Dr*. Barnard.

13 10.

13 10. *Finds Sense in* * Br---*Charms* in *Lady* † G---e.

* The late Sir *William Brownlow*. † *Grace*, the late Lady *Grace Pierrepoint*.

15 3. Colon----Mr. *Lee*.

4. Horoscope, *Dr*. Barnard.

17 Squirt----*Dr*. Barnard's *Man*.

CANTO III.

Pag. Ver.

18 4. COLON---*Mr*. Lee.

6. *And* * S----*Works*.

* *Salmon*, a late Quack Doctor, and indefatigable Scribbler.

20 6. Horoscope } *Dr*. Bernard.
14. Magus. }

10. *Tyro*'s Apprentices.

24. *Diasenna* ; either Mr. *Dare* an Apothecary, or according to others, Mr. Figge, late Master of the Apothecary's Company.

24 4. For * S----rs *has the Seal and* † Nassau *reigns*.

* *Somers*, the Lord *Somers*, late Lord Chancellor.

4. *Nassau*, the late King *WILLIAM*.

21. *Colocynthis*, Mr. *Baron*, an *Apothecary*.

25 6. *Russel*, Mr. a famous *Undertaker*, or *Upholder*.

27 24. *Ascarides*, Mr. *Bridges* and Mr. *Parret*, two *Apothecaries*.

CAN-

CANTO IV.

Pag. Ver.

32 1. FRequented *Theatre* : The *Playhouse in Drury-Lane*, near *Covent-Garden*.

5. *Bently*, a late Bookseller in *Great Russel-Street*.

6. *Briscoe*, another Bookseller, late of *Covent-Garden*, and formerly Mr. *Bently*'s Prentice.

11. *When* * Bur---ss *deafens all the list'ning Press*.

* Dr. *Burgess*, a famous *Presbyterian* Preacher.

13. *Mysterious* † F---n

‖ Dr. *Freeman*, late Rector of *Covent-Garden*.

43 21. }
29. } Mirmillo : Dr. *Gibbons* of *King-Street, Covent-Garden*.

33 6. Askaris : Mr. *Parrot*, an Apothecary.

27. Querpo : Dr. *How*.

34 7. Carus : Dr. *Tyson*, Physician of *Bedlam*.

35 4. * M---*Works entire, and endless Reams of* ‖ B---m.

* Dr. *Henry Moor*'s Works.

† B---m, Mr. *Bloom* the late Editor of Books by Subscription.

5. ----*neglected* C---s : Dr. *Collins*.

6. } Carus : Dr. *Tyson*.
8. } ----

9. } Umbra : Dr. *Cole*.
13. } -----

23. * C---*a* Lycurgus, *and a* Phocion † R---

* Sir *Henry Colt*, late Member of Parliament for *Westminster*.

† Mr. *Anthony Rowe*.

Pag. Ver.

24. Horoſcope: Dr. *Bernard.*

36 1. Vagellius: Sir *Barth. Shore,* a late Lawyer, famous for Declamation.

9. * Or---d *ſuſpected,* † D---b *innocent.*

* The Earl of *Orford.*

† The late Sir *Charles Duncomb.*

36 24. *Arms meet with Arms,* &c. Verſes quoted out of Dr. *Blackmore*'s King *Arthur,* and Prince *Arthur.*

37 22. *Read* * W---, *conſider* † D---n *well.*

* Mr. *Wycherly,* a Poet famous for ſolid Wit and Senſe.

† Mr. *Dryden,* a late Poet, who will ever be famous for good Verſification.

25. *If* * D---'s *ſprightly Muſe.*

* The late Earl of *Dorſet.*

29. ----*Th' immortal Brows of* * A---n.

* Mr. *Addiſon,* a famous Poet bred at *Oxford.*

38 1. *Tuneful* C---ve: Mr. *Congreve,* a Poet principally famous for his *Paſtorals* and *Dramatick* Writings.

6. St---: The late Mr. *Stepney.*

7. P---: Mr. *Matthew Prior,* a Poet.

10. Sequana: the *Seine,* the River that runs through *Paris.*

17. M---ue's, *Montague,* Lord *Halifax.*

40 10. *And each brave* * Churchill of the Galaxy.

* A high, nice, and juſt Complement the Author pays to the Duke of *Marlborough*'s Daughter.

42 19. *Sir* Scrape-Quill----Any Upſtart in the City, or at Court.

23. Spa-

Pag. Ver.

23. Spadillio: A Footman, who has got an Estate: I suppose the Author means Mr. *A---M---.*

43 6. *Shall for a* H---, *a greater* M---*find.*

* *Hesse*, the late Prince of *Hesse Darmstadt.*

† *Mordaunt*, the Earl of *Peterborow* and *Monmouth*, who took *Barcelona*, after the Death of the Prince of *Hesse.*

CANTO V.

Pag. Ver.

44 8. MIRMILLO, Dr. *Gibbons.*

45 19. *Have I made* * S---th, *and* ‖ Sh---ck *disagree?*

* Dr. *South*, Prebendary of *Westminster*, and Dr. ‖ *Sherlock*, late Dean of St. *Paul*'s, and Master of the *Temple*, who wrote against one another about the TRINITY; and so managed the Controversy that the Publick were of Opinion, That the first proved, there is but one GOD; and the other, That there are Three. The Dispute was ridiculed in a Ballad, to the Tune of, *A Soldier and a Sailor*, &c. and which begins thus,

A Dean and Prebendary,
Had once a new Vagary, &c.

21. F---*son*, Ferguson, the famous *Plot Monger.*

46 21. *Let* ‖ P--- *speak*, and * V---k write.

‖ The Earl of *Peterborow.*

* Mr. *Vanbruck*: A Gentleman much cry'd up for his Dramatick Pieces, when the *Dispensary* was first writ; but who has since turned his Genius to *Architecture.*

Pag. Ver.

46 25. *Had* * C----h *printed nothing of his own.*

26. *He had not been the* ‖ S----fold *of the Town.*

* Dr. *Colbatch.*

‖ *Saffold*, a celebrated Empirick, whose Bills were formerly set up in all Publick *Diuretick* Places in *London* and *Westminster*, to the great Comfort and Entertainment of idle Country-Folks.

47 1. *Had* ‖ W---*never aim'd in Verse to please.*

Mr. ‖ *Westley*, a Divine, who has wrote a great deal of *Holy Doggrel.*

2. Ogilby's : Mr. *Ogilby* would have perhaps got some Reputation, if he had aspired no higher than *Reynard the Fox :* But having ventur'd to translate in Verse the sublimest *Latin* Poets, his Name will, as long as the *English* Tongue lives, signify a *Poetaster.*

8. *And to a* * B---ly *'tis we owe a* ‖ B---le.

* Dr. *Bently*, Keeper of the Royal Library.

‖ *Charles Boyle*, the present Earl of *Orrery.*

Towards the close of the last Century, There arose a Dispute between those two Gentlemen, about the Epistles of *Phalaris*, which was maintain'd with a great deal of *Urbanity* and *good Manners* on one Side, and with equal *Sufficiency* and *Pedantry* on the other Side.

19. Mirmillo : Dr. *Gibbons.*

47 9. -----

19. -----

48 22. Querpo : Dr. *How.*

24. *By* Mulciber *the Mayor of* Bromingham.

Every one knows that *Mulciber* was one of the Heathen Gods, otherwise called *Vulcan* ; But 'tis

Pag. Ver.

'tis the Opinion of many, that our Poet means here Mr. *Th---Fol---* a Lawyer of notable Parts.

49 13. } Querpo : Dr. *How*.
25. } -----

19. Querpoides : Dr. *How's* Son.

26. Carus : Dr. *Tyson*.

51 20. *That* * P---k's *Worth, and* ‖ O---'s *Valour tells*

* The Earl of *Pembroke*.

‖ The Duke of *Ormond*.

21. *How Truth in* * B---, *how in* ‖ C---sh *reigns*.

* *Burnet* : The late Bishop of *Sarum*.

† *Cavendish* : The Duke of *Devonshire*.

51 24. *If* ‖ W---*plead, or* * S--- *or* † O---ly *preach*.

‖ Sir *Francis Winnington*.

* Dr. *South*.

† Dr. *Only*, Minister at St. *Margaret's*.

28. Stentor, Dr. *Goodall*, of the *Charter-house*.

52 1. Machaon, Sir *Tho. Millington*, President of the College of Physicians.

54 6. Stentor, Dr. *Goodall*.

7. Carus, Dr. *Tyson*.

8. Colon : Mr. *Lee*.

Sertorius : A Physician.

12. Chiron : Dr. *Gill*.

Talthibius. Another Physician.

16. Psylas : Dr. *Chamberlayne*, Man-Midwife.

54 29. Hermes. A Physician.

I 3 55 3

55 3. Trismegists. Two other Physicians.
19. Stentor : Dr. *Goodall.*
20. Querpo : Dr. *How.*
4. Querpoides : Dr. *How*'s Son.
57 15. The Heroe : Dr. *How.*

CANTO VI.

Pag. Ver.
58 6. *AND borrow* * C---le's *Shape,* and ‖ G---'s *Air.*
* *Cecile :* The late Countess of *Salisbury.*
‖ The Dutchess of *Grafton.*
7. *Her Eyes like* * R . . . gh's *their Beams dispense.*
* The Countess of *Ranelagh.*
58 8. *With* * C---ll's *Bloom, and* ‖ B . . . . ey's *Innocence.*
* *Churchill,* one of the Duke of *Marlborough*'s Daughters.
‖ The Countess of *Berkley.*
12. Machaon : Sir *Tho. Millington.*
59 5. } Celsus : Dr. *Bateman,* a Physician.
9. } . . . . . .
18. Strimonian *Squadron : i. e.* The *Cranes.*
19. *The Delegates :* } Dr. *Bateman.*
27. *Heav'nly Guide.* }
59 7. Hygeia, *the* Goddess *Health.*
8. Celsus : Dr. *Bateman.*
20. *Copious* M. . . . : Dr. *Moore.*
64 7. Celsus : Dr. *Bateman.*

Guiacum

Pag.	Ver.	
64	4.	Guiacum: Mr. *Hobbs*, Surgeon.
	13.	Celsus: Dr. *Bateman.*
	30.	*Bless'd* Harvey: The late famous Dr. *Harvey*, who compleated the Discovery of the *Circulation of the Blood.*
66	8.	Celsus: } Dr. *Bateman.*
	26.	Delegate: } Dr. *Bateman.*
67	9.	Olivia } Whoever has the least Knowledge of the Town and *Beau Monde*, will easily know where to fix these three *fictitious Names.*
68	7.	Rufilla: }
	9.	Cælia: }
68	1.	Hygeia: Health.
	24.	Willis: Dr. *Willis.*
69	1.	Wharton, Bates, *and* Glisson: Three Doctors of Physick.
	5.	*Your* Charge: Dr. *Bateman.*
	7.	*Matchless* Atticus: The Lord *Somers*, then Lord Chancellor.
	8.	Great *NASSAU*: The late KING *WILLIAM.*
71	3.	*Would* Phœbus, *or his* * G----le, *but inspire.*
		* *Granville*, the present Lord *Lansdowne.*

VERSES omitted in the late Editions of the *Dispensary*.

CANTO I. Page 3. after *Impudence to* S——e, add

WHY *Atticus* polite, *Brutus* severe,
Why *Me*.....*n* muddy, *M*......*gue* why clear.

Ibid. Page 7. after *and thus went on.*

Sometimes among the *Caspian* Cliffs I creep,
Where solitary Bats and Swallows sleep.
Or if some Cloyster's Refuge I implore,
Where holy Drones o'er dying Tapers snore;
Still *Nassau*'s Arms a soft Repose deny,
Keep me awake, and follow where I fly.

Since he has bless'd the weary World with Peace,
And with a Nod has bid *Bellona* cease:
I sought the Covert of some peaceful Cell,
Where silent Shades in harmless Raptures dwell;
That Rest might past Tranquillity restore,
And Mortal never interrupt me more.

Canto II. Page 11. after *unrelenting Storm*, add

Then ſhe: Alas! how long in vain have I
Aim'd at thoſe noble Ills the Fates deny:
Within this Iſle for ever muſt I find
Diſaſters to diſtract my reſtleſs Mind?
Good *T*....*n*'s Celeſtial Piety
At laſt has rais'd him to the Sacred See.
So....*rs* does ſick'ning Equity reſtore,
And helpleſs Orphans are opreſs'd no more.
Pem....*ke* to *Britain* endleſs Bleſſing brings;
He ſpoke; and Peace clap'd her Triumphant Wings:
Great *O*....*nd* ſhines illuſtriouſly bright
With Blazes of Hereditary Light.
The noble Ardour of a Royal Fire
Inſpires the generous Breaſt of *D*....*re*.
And *M*....*d* is active to defend
His Country with the Zeal he loves his Friend.
Like *Leda*'s radiant Sons divinely clear,
P....*land* and *J*....*ſey* deck'd in Rays appear,
To gild by turns the *Gallick* Hemiſphere.
Worth in Diſtreſs is rais'd by *M*....*gue*,
Auguſtus liſtens if *Mæcenas* ſue.
And *Ve*....*n*'s Vigilance no ſlumber takes,
Whilſt Faction peeps abroad, and Anarchy awakes.

Canto

Canto III. Page 21. after *discern each hour*, add

Thou that would'st lay whole *States* and *Regions* waste,
Sooner than we thy *Cormorants* should fast;

Ibid. Page 24. after *Spring and Fall*, add

But now late Jars our Practices detect,
For Mines, when once discover'd, lose th' Effect.
Dissentions, like small Streams, are first begun,
Scarce seen they rise, but gather as they run:
So Lines that from their Parallel decline,
More they advance, the more they still dis-joyn.
Tis therefore my Advice, in haste we send,
And beg the Faculty to be our Friend.
As he revolving stood to say the rest,
Rough *Colocynthis* thus his Rage exprest.

Canto IV. Page 37. after *amorous Fire*, add

The *Tyber* now no gentle *Gallus* sees,
But smiling *Thames* enjoys her *No- - - -by's*.

Canto V. Page 52. after *Foes, or die*, add

What Stentor offer'd was by most approv'd;
But sev'ral Voices sev'ral Methods mov'd.
At length th'adventrous *Heroes* all agree
T' expect the Foe, and act offensively.

Into

Into the Shop their bold *Batallions* move,
And what their Chief commands the reſt approve.
Down from the *Walls* they tear the *Shelves* in haſte,
Which on their Flank for palliſades are plac'd.
And then, behind the Compter rang'd they ſtand,
Their Front ſo well ſecur'd obey Command.
And now the Scouts the adverſe Hoſt deſcry,
Blue Aprons in the Air for Colours fly:
With unreſiſted Force they urge their Way,
And find the Foe embattel'd in Array.

Ibid. Page 56. after *wink at Hereſy*, add

Faith ſtand unmov'd thro' *S- - - -fleet's* Defence,
And *L- - - -k* for Myſtery abandon Senſe.

A Con-

A Continuation of the KEY.

Mirmillo,	Dr. *Gibbons*
Stentor,	Dr. *Goodall*
Bard,	Sir *Richard Blackmore*
Celſus,	Dr. *Bateman*
Machaon,	Dr. *Millington*
Atticus,	Lord *Chancellor* Somers
Carus,	Dr. *Tyſon*
Querpo,	Dr. *How*
Brutus,	Ld. Ch. Juſt. *Holt*
Horoſcope *and* Magus,	Dr. *Barnard*
Colocynthis	*Dare*, an Apothecary
Vagellius	Serjeant *Darnell*
Colon	*Lee* an Apothecary
S----,	*Sands*
M--- -n,	*Methwin*
Br----w,	*Brownlow*
Sa----ds,	Dr. *Salmonds*
Aſcarides	*Bridges* and *Parrot*
C----s,	Dr. *Collins*
Scribarius,	Dr. *Lyſter*
Pſylas,	Dr. *Woodward.*
C . . . . h,	*Colebatch* Chirurgeon
O . . . . y	*Onely*, Parſon of St. *Martins.*
A . . . . on,	*Addiſon*
Umbra,	Dr. *Gould*
C . . . . t,	Sir *H. Colt*
R . . . . ,	*Row*
C . . . . ls,	*Cecills*
Hygea,	The *Goddeſs of* Health
Delegate *and* Celſus,	Dr. *Garth*
P . . . . ps,	*Phillips*
Guiacum	Dr. *Hobbs*
Ch . . . . ll's	*Churchill's*
Mulciber,	*Thomas Foley*
Chiron,	Dr. *Gill*
Lucina,	Dr. *Chamberlayn*
Pauſanias,	a Play by *Norton.*

FINIS.

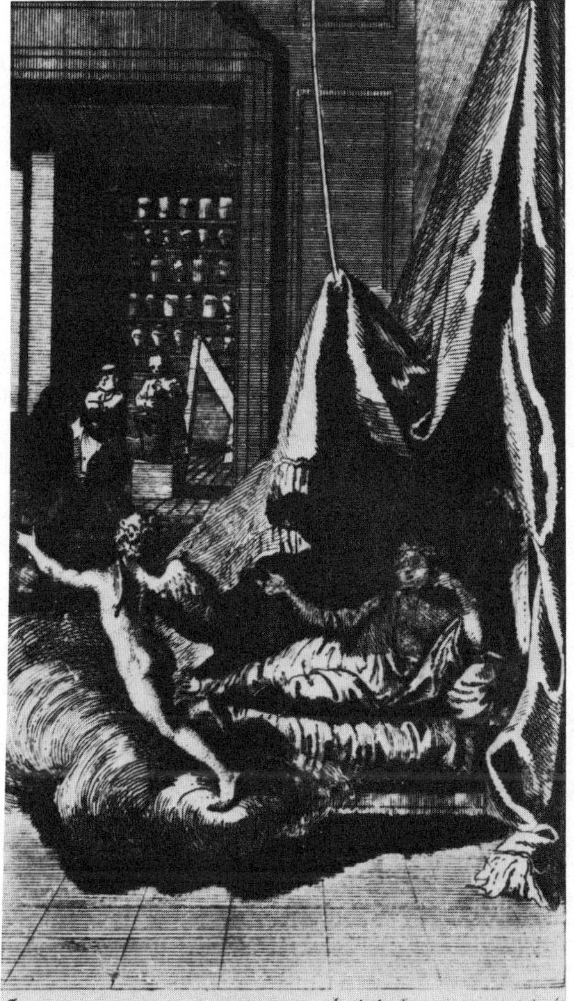

Can. 1. *Lud. du Guernier inv. et Sculp.*

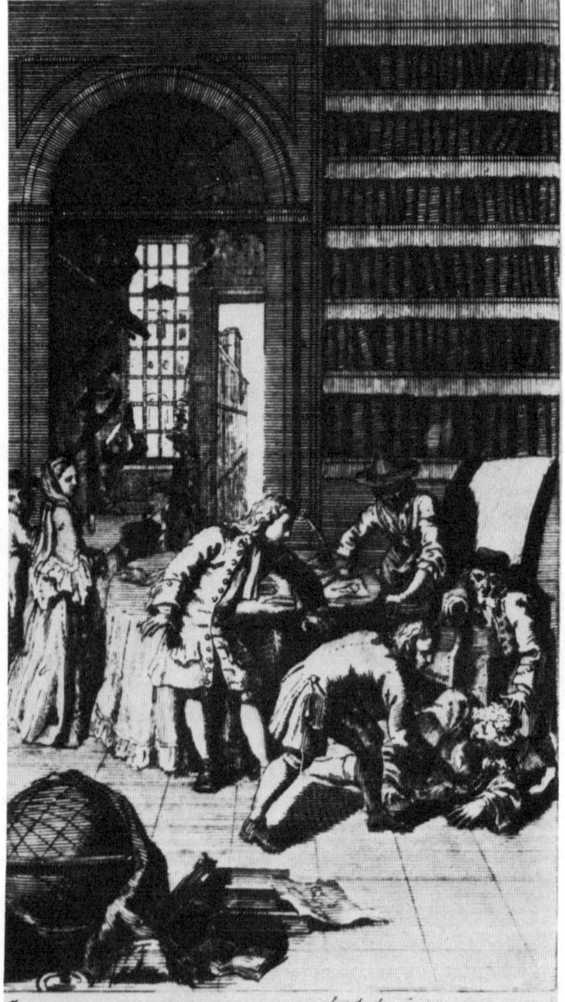

Can. 2.

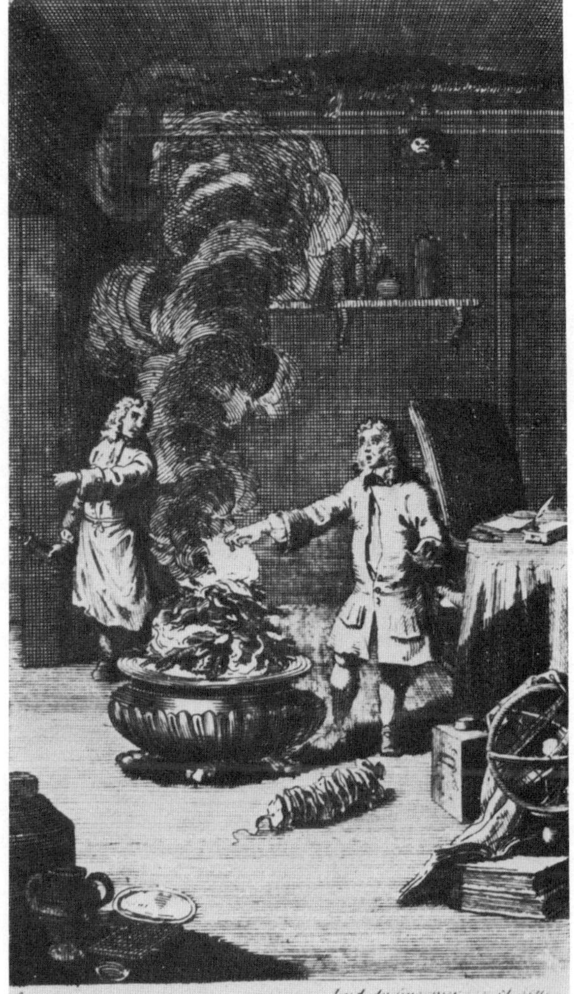
Can. 3
Lud. du

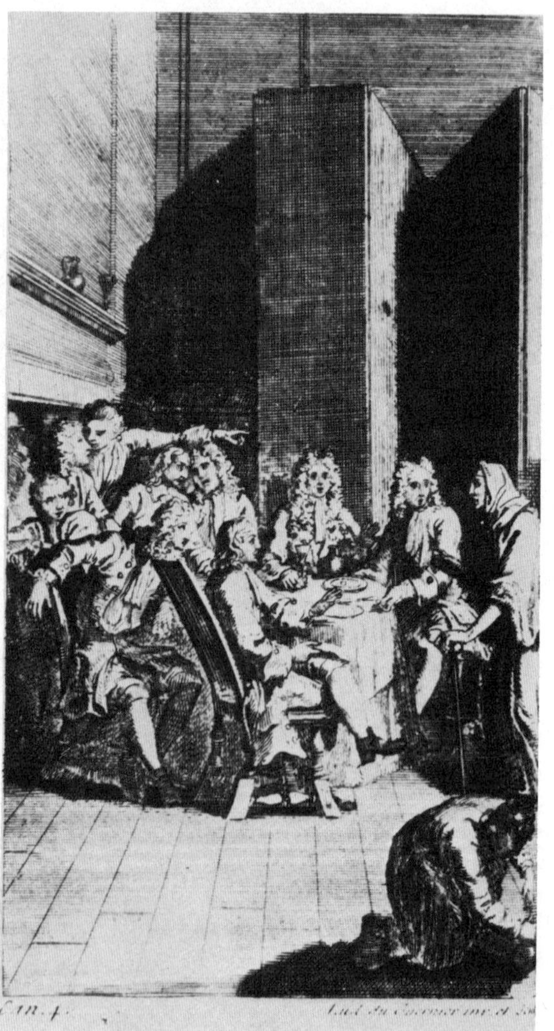

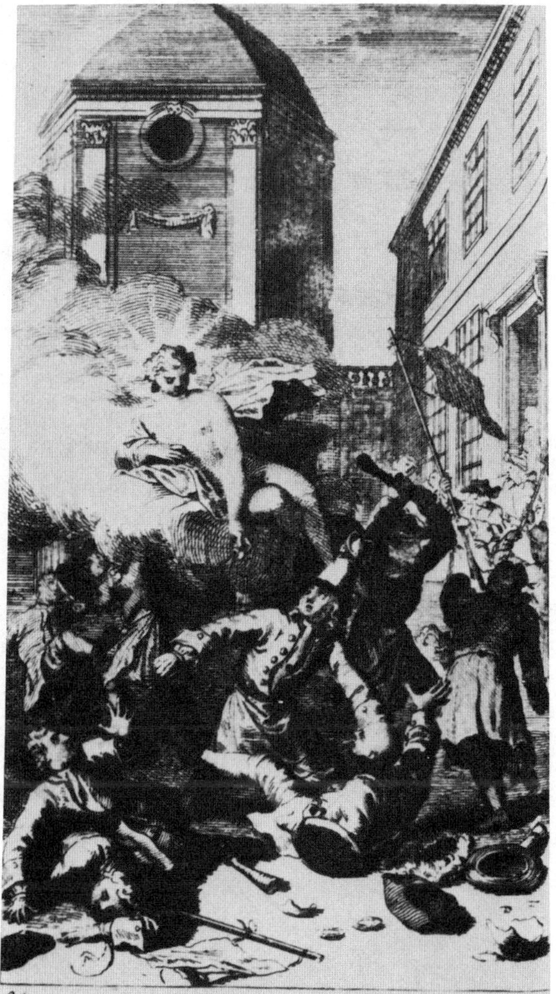
Can. 5.

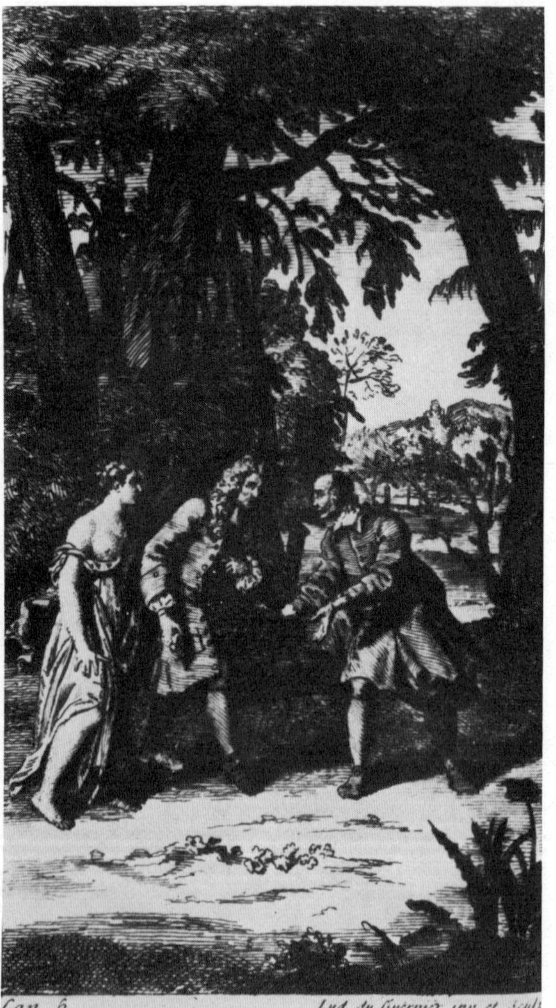

Can. 6. *Lud. du Guernier inv. et Sculp*

A

Short Account

OF THE

PROCEEDINGS

OF THE

College of Physicians, *London*,

In relation to the

SICK POOR

Of the said

CITY and SUBURBS thereof,

With the Reasons which have induced the College to make Medicines for them at the Intrinsick Value.

LONDON, Printed in the Year 1697.

THIS Following Treatise [A short Account of the Proceedings of the College of Physicians, &c.] having been considered and examined by the Committee of the said College, they thought fit to recommend it to the President and Censors to be published.

IMPRIMATUR.

Datum ex Ædibus Collegii nostri in Comitiis Censoriis Junii 11. 1697.

Tho. Millington, *Praeses.*
Tho. Burwell,
Rich. Torless,
W. Dawes,
Tho. Gill, } Censors.

A Short Account OF THE PROCEEDINGS OF THE College of Physicians, *London*, In relation to the Sick Poor, &c.

SINCE it hath been the fate of many good Undertakings though in themselves highly beneficial to the Publick, to miscarry and come to nothing, not so much by the *open opposition* of interessed and designing Persons, as by their *private insinuations* and *misrepresentations*, whereby they prepossess the People to their own great hurt and damage: That the like misfortune may not befal the charitable Design now set on foot by the *College of Physicians, LONDON*, for the Relief of the *Poor Sick* in and about this great City and Suburbs, We have thought it necessary to give a short historical account of the Rise and Progress of this matter, whereby we hope it will appear, That this Undertaking, as it was several years since begun (before there were any differences or misunderstandings either amongst our selves, or with the Apothecaries) upon no other ground but the commiseration of the deplorable condition of the Poor Sick, (especially poor House-keepers) not usually taken care of by the Parishes; so also that the same hath been ever since carried on with the same honest intention: And we doubt not but a work so advantagious to the Sick Poor, and so honourable to this City, will in the same manner be shortly finish'd and brought to its utmost perfection.

To omit therefore what has in former times been attempted of this nature by our Predecessors (of whose early Charity we have several Instances recorded in our Annals) the first step we find tending directly to this purpose is a Vote of the College in their publick Meeting, *July* 28. 1687. to this effect: "It was this day "appointed and ordained by the *Unanimous Vote* of the College, "That all the Members thereof, whether Fellows, Candidates, or "Licentiates of the said College, shall give their advice *gratis* "to all their sick neighbouring Poor, when desired, within the "City of *London*, or seven miles round.

This Order being carried by several of the Members of the College to the Lord Mayor and Court of Aldermen, They (*Aug.* 23. 1687.) did by Dr. *Betts*, one of our Elects, return the College Thanks for this their charitable Order; with this further request to the College, That they would explain themselves, as to whom they meant by *Poor*? which they did, by declaring, That all those should be esteemed *Poor*, that brought Certificates under the hand of the Rector, Vicar or Curate of the Parish wherein they dwelt, of their being such.

An account of this was by the respective Aldermen sent to each Ward. But partly by the industry of some Persons, with whose private Gain it was not so consistent, and especially by reason of the high Prices of Medicines above the purchace of Poor House-keepers, it was for that time stifled. Which the College perceiving, and desirous that so good an Intention to so many poor People might not be frustrated, several methods for the removing this obstruction were

were propoſed at their general Meetings, as, The expending all the Fines of the College in providing Phyſick for the Poor, and the like: And at laſt they came to this Reſolution, (which was paſt into an Order, *Aug.* 13. 1688.) *viz.*

The College having conſidered that the Charitable Vote which formerly paſſed for preſcribing to the Poor gratis, *hath not had the effect intended, by reaſon of the great Prices they are obliged to pay for their Medicines, have this day unanimouſly voted, That the Laboratory of the College be forthwith fitted up for preparing Medicines for the Poor, and alſo the room adjoyning for a Repoſitory.* And the College further gave a power to thoſe Members who would ſubſcribe to this Charitable Work, to chooſe a Committee from among themſelves who ſhould order what Compoſitions and Simples ſhould be kept at the College for the benefit of the Poor, and manage the whole affair as they thought fit.

It was expected that upon this Order the Apothecaries (rather than the College ſhould make Medicines themſelves) would have ſo far concurred in this Charitable Work, as to have born their part therein: And that as we had freely offered our pains to preſcribe for the Poor for nothing, ſo they would have given them *their* pains alſo, in furniſhing them with neceſſary Medicines at the Intrinſick Value, or at leaſt for ſome ſmall Profit. But inſtead of that, ſeveral amongſt them ſet themſelves by all the art and induſtry they were capable of, to fruſtrate the whole deſign; and finding no method ſo promiſing as to ſtir up a party among our ſelves to oppoſe our proceedings, they fell to intrigueing with ſeveral of our own Members, who were too eaſily lured off to ſerve the Apothecaries intereſt, for their own private advantage. And from this cauſe, as we have too much reaſon to believe, have chiefly ſprung the unhappy Differences that are ſtill fomented among us.

But notwithſtanding all the diſcouragements we met with from thoſe of our own Members, who contrary to all the Obligations of Honour and Conſcience, conſtantly diſcovered to our Adverſaries whatſoever paſſed in the College relating to this deſign, and expoſed to them the Names of ſuch as were Promoters thereof, that they might be kept out, as far as in them lay, from all Patients where they ſhould be propoſed, and themſelves brought in; Theſe and ſeveral other difficulties were (though after a conſiderable time intervening) at last broke through, and the College proceeded to enforce their former Order by another of the 18*th*. *March* 1694. to this effect: *Whereas in the year* 1687. *there was an Order made by the unanimous consent of the College, obliging every Member thereof to give his Advice* gratis *in their respective Parishes in the Cities of* London *and* Westminster, *and Suburbs thereof, to all Poor Sick, as should be recommended to them for such by the Rector, Vicar or Curate of the said Parishes by Certificate under their Hands; which said Order was presented to the City: Now we judge it necessary that the said Order be again presented to the Lord Mayor, Court of Aldermen and Common Council, and do hereby again require strict Obedience from all our Members to the aforesaid Order.* And a Committee was then chosen by the College to take care of the managing this matter to the best advantage of the designed Charity (consisting of the Elects, Censors and 8. Fellows, whereof 5. to be a Committee.)

This Order was accordingly presented to the Lord Mayor, Court of Aldermen and Common Council, *June* 18. 1695. Upon which the Common Council did nominate, appoint and choose Sir *John Moor*, Sir *William Hedges* and Sir *Jos. Smart*, Aldermen; Mr. *Dorvile*, Mr. *Ballow*, Mr. *Egglestone*, Sir *Edmund Wiseman*, Mr. *Richer*, and Mr. *Palfreman*, Commoners, (whereof any one of the said Aldermen, and two of the said Commoners, to be a Committee) to return the Thanks of that Court to the College of Physicians for such their Order, and with them to consult how to improve the advantage proposed by the said College for the relief of the said poor Inhabitants.

July 24*th*. The Committee of the City and College met, where the Thanks of the Lord Mayor, Court of Aldermen and Common Council, was returned to the College of Physicians for their Charitable Order.

The Committee of the College delivered in a List of the Names of all their Members, with the places where they lived, which was desired by the City to be printed.

Then the Committee of the City made several Proposals or Queries; as First, Who should be recommended as fitting objects of this Charity? Secondly, Who should be the Persons, that should make up the Physicians Prescriptions, in the several Wards and Parishes of the City? Thirdly, Who should price the Medicines prescribed by the Physicians Bills?

After

After which they with the College-Committee, passing over the first Proposal (which was sufficiently answered by the College's Order) proceeded to debate the second and third, and came to this Resolution, That some Apothecaries should be found out who should supply the Poor with Medicines at such Rates as should be adjudged reasonable by the Physicians, in or near the several Parishes; which the Committee of the City earnestly recommended to the Physicians to take care of, and promised that they would doe the same on their part.

Upon this the Committee of the College applyed themselves with great diligence to answer the said desire of the City-Committee, and after some time found out several honest and charitable Apothecaries, who very cheerfully and readily embraced the offer, and at the solicitation of the Physicians, entred into this following Subscription: *We whose names are here underwritten are willing to furnish the Poor, within our respective Parishes, with Medicines at such Rates as the Committee of Physicians shall judge reasonable. Witness our hands.* Which subscription we have now by us, but for the Subscribers sakes, do not divulge their Names.

When the Committee of the College had got a sufficient number of Apothecaries, to furnish all the Wards of *London*, they acquainted the Committee of the City therewith, requesting them at the same time, that they would for their Encouragement, endeavour to have an Act passed in the Common Council, to excuse these Charitable Apothecaries from any troublesome Office.

Then the Committee of the City did desire the College-Committee to get a further Addition to their former Order, whereby the Churchwardens and Overseers of the Poor, or any of them, might as well as the Ministers, recommend by Certificate, fit Objects of Charity, as also that all hired Servants, and Apprentices to Handicrafts men, should be reckoned as Objects of Charity; which the Committee of the College promised to endeavour.

Now the College thought they had surmounted all Difficulties, and had attained their end: But the Apothecaries Company having got knowledge of our Meeting with a Committee of the City, did not only draw up and present a Paper to the Committee of the City tending wholly to frustrate the charitable ends of our design, which was sufficiently answered Article by Article, by the Committee

mittee of the College, Copies of both which are hereafter inserted; but also hearing that the Committee of Physicians had gotten Apothecaries enough to supply this Charity, they were extreamly alarmed, and presently called a Hall, wherein partly by threatning to impose upon them the most troublesome and expensive Offices of their Company, and partly by charging them upon this compliance with the Physicians, with breach of their Oaths to their Company, they affrighted most of these Apothecaries from this undertaking, as if their Oath obliged them, Not to do any thing charitably.

September the 4th. 1695. The College made such addition to their Order as the City-Committee had desired. At which Meeting the College did likewise approve and confirm all that had been done by their Committee, giving them thanks for the care and trouble they had already taken, and desiring them to proceed and perfect this charitable Work: owning and declaring all that the Committee had done to be the Act of the College, and not the Act of Six or Seven men, as some had industriously though falsely given out, and that the College would accordingly stand by their Committee in what they had done.

At the next Meeting of the Committees, the addition by the College to their former Order desired by the City-Committee, was delivered to them, who were much pleased therewith. Then they proceeded to consider who should price the Medicines. And the College-Committee was content (because they would avoid every thing that might obstruct this designed Charity) that the Master and Wardens of the Apothecaries Company should do it every Year, and afterwards bring it to the President and Censors of the College for their Approbation: but even this was also opposed by the Apothecaries Company.

Thus it appearing that the Apothecaries were resolved to obstruct this Charity in every particular, the City-Committee ask'd the Physicians then present, Whether their College would provide Medicines for the Poor at reasonable Rates, if the Apothecaries should continue to refuse so to do? To which they answered, That they believed, rather than so Charitable a design should fail, the College would undertake it; and promis'd that they would propose it at their next publick College-meeting.

Hereupon

Hereupon the City-Committee being fully satisfied with the Physicians Answers to their Proposals, and with their sincerity in transacting this whole affair with them, as also that the methods offered by them were the most proper for obtaining the end proposed, drew up a Report accordingly, of the whole matter, which the Chairman Sir *William Hedges* offered to read at the next Common Council: but some affair that required a quicker dispatch intervening, it was put off for that time; and this happening at the latter end of the year, the Common Council was not long after of course dissolved, and another chosen, in which several of the then Committee were left out; which probably was the cause that this Report was never after called for.

The matter resting thus, and the College being in expectation to hear from the City, they did nothing further in it till *Decemb.* 22. *1696.* when a Proposition was made in the publick College for a Subscription by the Fellows, Candidates and Licentiates, for carrying on this Charity, which being therein approved, (about nine or ten only dissenting) a Subscription to the effect following was immediately made.

W*Hereas the several Orders of the College of Physicians* London, *for prescribing Medicins* gratis *to the Poor Sick of the Cities of* London *and* Westminster, *and parts adjacent, as also the Proposals made by the said College to the Lord Mayor, Court of Aldermen and Common Council of* London, *in pursuance thereof, have hitherto been ineffectual, for that no method hath been taken to furnish the Poor with Medicins for their Cure at low and reasonable rates: We therefore whose names are here underwritten, Fellows or Members of the said College, being willing effectually to promote so great a Charity, by the Counsel and good liking of the President and College declared in their* Comitia, *hereby (to wit, each of us severally and apart, and not the one for the other of us) do oblige our selves to pay to* Dr. Thomas Burwel, *Fellow and Elect of the said College, the sum of Ten Pounds apiece of Lawful Money of* England, *by such proportions, and at such times as to the major part of the Subscribers hereto shall seem most convenient: Which Money when received by the said* Dr. Thomas Burwel,

Burwel, *is to be by him expended in preparing and delivering Medicins to the Poor at their intrinsick Value, in such manner, and at such Times, and by such Orders and Directions, as by the major part of the Subscribers hereto, shall in Writing be hereafter appointed and directed for that purpose. In Witness whereof we have hereunto set our Hands and Seals this Twenty Second Day of* December, *1696.*

Tho. Millington, *Præses.*
Tho. Burwell, *Elect and Censor.*
Sam. Collins, *Elect.*
Edw. Browne, *Elect.*
Rich. Torless, *Elect and Censor.*
Edw. Hulse, *Elect.*
Tho. Gill, *Censor.*
Will. Dawes, *Censor.*
Jo. Hutton.
Rob. Brady.
Hans Sloane.
Rich. Morton.
John Hawys.
Ch. Harel.
Rich. Robinson.
Joh. Bateman.
Walter Mills.
Dan. Coxe.
Henry Sampson.
Thomas Gibson.
Charles Coodall.
Edm. King.
Sam. Garth.
Barnh. Soame.
Denton Nicholas.
Joseph Gaylard.
John Woollaston.
Steph. Hunt.
Oliver Horseman.
Rich. Morton, *Jun.*
David Hamilton.
Hen. Morelli.
Walter Harris.
William Briggs.
Th. Colladon.
Martin Lister.
Jo. Colbatch.
Bernard Connor.
W. Cockburn.
J. le Feure.
P. Sylvestre.
Cha. Morton.

This

THIS Inſtrument being thus ſubſcribed by the Preſident, the Cenſors, all the Elects, but two, moſt of the Senior Fellows, and ſeveral of the Candidates and Licentiates; a College was called, That a Grant might be forthwith made by way of Leaſe to the Subſcribers, of the Laboratory, and other Rooms and conveniencies neceſſary for executing the intended charitable deſign. Which, notwithſtanding the oppoſition of ſome few, was by a very great majority granted, and afterwards ſealed in open College. And now the Laboratory, Repoſitory, &c. are preparing with all imaginable expedition, that ſo the benefit of the preſent ſeaſon for making all ſorts of neceſſary Medicines for the uſe of the Sick Poor may not be loſt, but that we may be in a condition ſhortly to receive, make up, and diſtribute, all ſuch Bills and Preſcriptions as ſhall be directed to the Repoſitory by ſuch Phyſicians as have been ſo charitable as to ſubſcribe to this Undertaking for the benefit of their Poor Sick Neighbours.

Here follow the ANSWERS offered by the Apothecaries to the Propoſals of the City-Committee, with the Phyſicians Reply thereunto.

ANSWERS humbly offered by the Society of Apothecaries, to the Propoſals made by the Worſhipful the Committee appointed by Common Council to treat with the Phyſicians in relation to the Poor.

THAT in purſuance of your Worſhips Directions, We the Maſter, Wardens and Aſſiſtants of the ſaid Society have maturely conſidered the Propoſals to us made. And in the firſt place crave leave to return our Thanks and due acknowledgment to this Committee, for communicating the ſaid matters and Propoſals of the Phyſicians to us, and do moſt willingly take this opportunity to declare, That as we eſteem it our principal Glory to be Members of this great and honourable City, ſo we ſhall be ever ready to contribute to the utmoſt of our Power to the Honour and Welfare thereof, or any the Members depending thereon. And to that end,

C To

To the First Proposal,

Who may be fittest persons to recommend the Objects of Charity?

WE take it, That the Minister, Churchwardens, and Overseers of the Poor in each Parish are the most fit, as best knowing the Poor and their necessity.

To the Second,

Who shall administer the Physick, &c?

WE do with submission think it most convenient, That it be left to every Parish from time to time to make use of what Apothecary they please, being a Freeman, within their own Parish, either one or more, according to the smalness or largeness thereof. And in case any Parish be without an Apothecary, then to take any neighbouring Freeman as they shall think fit.

To the Third,

Who shall price the Medicines delivered for the use of the Poor?

WE are humbly of opinion, That every man in his own way is best able to make his own Bill, and hope it will be sufficient satisfaction in this point, that we undertake, That all our Members shall use the greatest moderation possible; and in case any dispute arise, That then as to all Medicines delivered to the use of such Poor for whom the Churchwardens of each Parish shall be obliged to pay, the price shall be regulated to the intrinsick value of every Medicine by the Master and Wardens for the time being.

And for the better promoting so good a work, the Master, Wardens and Assistants of this Company do further offer, not only from time to time, to sell such Poor their Medicines when prescribed by a Physician at their intrinsick value, but (if it may be acceptable and approved of by an Order of this Honourable Court) *They will*, being thereto summoned by the Churchwardens or Overseers of any Parish in the absence of a Physician, and until one can be called in, *give them all the assistance they are capable of, by administring such Remedies as may be necessary, and that without reward or payment either for Pains or Medicines.* *The*

The Opinion of the Committee of the College of Physicians concerning the Anſwer *of the Apothecaries to the* Propoſals *made to them by the Worſhipful the Committee appointed by common Council to treat with the Phyſicians in relation to the Poor.*

TO the *Firſt Propoſal* we agree, *viz.* That the Miniſters, Churchwardens and Overſeers of the Poor of each Pariſh do recommend to the Phyſicians ſuch as they ſhall judge *Objects of Charity.*

To the *Second,* We think it moſt proper that the Common Council ſhould chuſe and appoint one or more Apothecaries, being Freemen, in each Pariſh or Ward, or any Neighbouring Apothecaries, if the Pariſh or Ward be without one; and that the Shops of ſuch Apothecaries be diſtinguiſh'd by ſome Inſcription, or other Mark, whereby they may be publickly known to the Phyſicians and Poor. Provided that no Apothecary be ſo appointed, nor continued in that imploy, who has done, or ſhall do any thing to prejudice or affront the City, or College of Phyſicians.

To the *Third,* We humbly conceive the Anſwer of the Apothecaries to be unſatisfactory, both in relation to the Almes-poor, and the Poor Inhabitants. Becauſe *Firſt,* For the *Alms-poor* it ſets no certain price upon their Medicines, but only allows, That if the Pariſh be diſſatisfied with the Rates of any Medicines, then upon application made to the Maſter and Wardens for the time being, thoſe Medicines for that time ſhall by them be rated at the intrinſick value, and ſo *toties quoties.* Now we judge this Branch of their Propoſal inconvenient to the Pariſhes for theſe Reaſons.

1. Becauſe the Churchwardens and Overſeers of the Poor being ſuppoſed to have no skill in the prices of Druggs and Medicines, cannot tell when they are well, or ill uſed therein, and conſequently know not when to complain.

2. Becauſe, If they did know, that yet ſuch frequent Applications (as it is poſſible there may be occaſion for) will be burthenſome to them; beſides that they may be unwilling to diſoblige their Neighbour Apothecaries by complaining of them.

3. Becauſe the Pariſhes cannot judge of the charge they are likely to be at upon the account of any Alms-Poor; But if either a certain Intrinſick Rate, or a moderate Profit be put upon Medicines, then all theſe inconveniences will be prevented.

But then *Secondly*, as for the *Poor Inhabitants*; it ſeems to us yet more neceſſary, that a certain moderate Price be from time to time (as Druggs ſhall conſiderably riſe or fall) put upon the Medicines, for theſe Reaſons.

1. Becauſe then ſuch Poor Patients may certainly know from the Phyſician the Price of any Medicines preſcribed for them, and ſo may be incouraged to take them. Whereas, if when they have a Bill from the Phyſician, they be ſtill left to the diſcretion of the Apothecary, the Price may prove too high for their Purſes, and they by this means be defeated of their Health, and the Charity intended.

2. Becauſe Poor Patients ignorant of the Price of the Medicines ordered for them, cannot tell when they are charitably uſed, or otherwiſe; and conſequently cannot complain of ſuch Apothecaries as ſhall exact upon them.

3. Becauſe the Apothecaries cannot then claſh amongſt themſelves, nor be cenſured by the Patients, upon the account that one ſells his Medicines dearer, and another cheaper; nor on the other hand can they agree together to raiſe their Medicines above the purchace of ordinary Poor Perſons, which they may otherwiſe inſenſibly do, and ſo make this publick Charity ineffectual by degrees.

4. We conceive this to be the beſt, if not the only way for the Apothecaries to demonſtrate to this City, That they are in earneſt (as no queſtion divers good men among them are) when they offer ſo freely to concur in this publick Charity. For whilſt they are left to their own Prices, it cannot be certain and clear, whether they are Charitable therein or no; but when the moderateneſs of their Rates is once fixed and certainly known to be ſo, their Charity will then be beyond ſuſpicion and contradiction.

In the mean time we are much miſrepreſented, if we be thought deſirous arbitrarily to fix the Prices of the Medicines: We are very willing

willing the Apothecaries ſhould do it themſelves: Only we think it highly neceſſary, both for their Credit, and the Service, as well as ſatisfaction of the City, That a Committee of the College (whom the like ſervice done the Publick both in the Armies and Navies demonſtrate to be competent Judges in this matter) ſhould agree to, and approve of thoſe Rates as moderate and charitable.

Wherefore we cannot but here expreſs our ſelves doubtful of the Apothecaries Sincerity in this matter, not only becauſe when this Propoſal was Seven Years ago offered to this City, they then made not the leaſt ſtep to comply therewith: but alſo becauſe at this time when ſeveral charitably diſpoſed Members of their Body offered to concurr with the College of Phyſicians in this good work, they did publickly in their Common Hall, threaten and intimidate them, pretending that any compliance herein with the Phyſicians in agreeing to the Rates of Medicines, would be againſt their Oaths. Whereas indeed it is ſo far from being ſo, that divers eminent perſons amongſt them, have for their profit in making Medicines for the Armies and Navies, ſeveral times, freely and without ſcruple conſented thereto. And we doubt not but if this City will ſo far influence the Apothecaries as to take off the terror they are now under, that there will appear a ſufficient number of charitable perſons amongſt them, very ready to ſerve in this Charity.

As to the Offer they make in *preſcribing Medicines to the Poor in the abſence of a Phyſician gratis*, if it may be approved by an Order of this Court: We are ſorry to meet with ſo clear a proof of their great Ambition to meddle with what belongs not to them, to ſet themſelves up for Phyſicians, and run themſelves into practice upon pretence of Charity to the Poor; for otherwiſe in the abſence of one Phyſician, there is no need of running to an Apothecary, ſince another in that caſe may be called: nor can we imagine why they ſhould be willing to give their Medicines *gratis*, whilſt they practiſe themſelves, and not ſo after a Phyſician is called in, if they did not intend practice thereby, and to hinder a Phyſicians being ſent for: this ſeems to be ſomething elſe than meer Charity. And for any Order of this Court to authoriſe them to practiſe upon the Poor, we conceive it wholly improper: for in Caſes of great and urgent neceſſity, not only any Apothecary, but any perſon that thinks he can do his poor ſick Neighbour good, may do it ſafely without any ſuch Order;

and

and for giving Licence to practise in other Cases, the Laws of the Land have setled that wholly in the College of Physicians. And therefore we desire that all Certificates for the Poor, be immediately directed and sent to the Physicians from the Officers of the Parishes, so that if any Physician shall find that an Apothecary without urgent necessity (as that Physician conceives,) has prescribed to the Poor Patient, he shall not be obliged to take care of that Patient.

Therefore upon the whole we humbly offer this as our opinion to this worshipful Committee, That the only way to make this publick Charity effectual is, That the Minister, Church-wardens and Overseers of the Poor, do recommend all charitable Objects immediately to the Physicians; That the Common Council do respectively chuse fitting persons in each Parish to be the known Apothecaries for the Poor; And that moderate and charitable Rates be fixed upon all Simples and compounded Medicines of the *London Dispensatory* by the Apothecaries (if they like it best) to be agreed to, and approved by a Committee of the Physicians, and known only to the Physicians, and themselves, and that only for the Publick benefit of the Poor of the City.

Lastly, we judge this proposal of fixing a certain Rate upon the Dispensatory-Medicines both so reasonable, and so absolutely necessary for the attaining the end designed in this publick Charity, that if the Apothecaries do refuse to agree thereto, rather than it should fail, we make no question but that the College of Physicians will undertake it themselves, and Print the Rate of their Medicines for the satisfaction of the Publick.

These *two* foregoing *Papers* were respectively delivered to the Committee of the City during the Treaty between them and the College in the year *1695*.

And now we desire leave from the foregoing History and Papers to make these following Observations.

1. That this great Charity was long ago set on foot, before any differences were arisen either amongst our Selves or with the Apothecaries as to these matters, and therefore is neither a rash nor hasty

hasty undertaking, nor entred upon with any intention to injure any body, or with any other sinister design, but out of meer Charity.

2. That it was at first *unanimously* undertaken, and the same reasons for it still continuing that at first moved us to it, those that now oppose it amongst our selves must necessarily do so for their private advantage, and the benefit of such as they are pleased to favour.

3. That all that was at first and for a great while after thought of in this Undertaking, was only to do our parts to the Sick Poor in prescribing to them *gratis*, not doubting then but the Apothecaries would do theirs, in concurring with us to afford them their Medicines at low and moderate Rates.

4. That to incourage them to do so, the Committee not only consented that the Master and Wardens themselves should price the Medicines (with the approbation of the College) but that such prices should be kept private, lest (as we supposed they chiefly fear'd) the rich coming thereby to understand at what Rates their Medicines might be afforded, should see clearly into their unreasonable Gains, and so bring down the excessive Rates of their Bills.

5. That the reasons which have induced the College to undertake the making up of Medicines for the Sick Poor, themselves, are as well their willingness to comply with the proposal hereof made by the City-Committee, as the necessity put upon them by the Apothecaries, who (as appears in the foregoing History) would not consent to any reasonable and satisfactory way of their own doing it. Besides that in their Answers to the City they did not take notice of any, but the meer *Alms-Poor*; whereas one main design of the College was to provide for *Poor Housekeepers*, and their Families that did not receive Alms.

6. And therefore if the Apothecaries come to any prejudice thereby at present, or in times to come, they must wholly blame themselves for it, and not the College, who were very far from intending them any harm by their Charity to others. But it is not reasonable that a work so highly commendable in it self, and so beneficial to the Poor Sick of this City and Suburbs, should [illegible] only to gratifie their humour and private interest.

7. However

7. However we hope this Undertaking will do the honeſt charitable Apothecaries no real injury, ſince we intend not to retail ſingle Medicines, but to write preſcriptions for the Sick Poor, to which every Phyſician ſo preſcribing ſhall underwrite the price of the Medicine, and the Patient to be at liberty to go either to any honeſt Apothecary that will faithfully make it up at that Rate, or to the College Repoſitory, where it will be ſo afforded. And certainly it will be no ſmall comfort to a Poor Patient to know preſently what his Phyſick will coſt him, and thereby to be freed from the dreadful apprehenſions of a chargeable and coſtly Bill, to be brought him afterwards by the Apothecary.

8. Upon the whole, As the Subſcribers being conſcious to themſelves of their Sincerity and Integrity in this Undertaking, reſt aſſured of the favour and applauſe of all good men: ſo if any of their Enemies ſhall be ſo void not only of Charity, but even of all Modeſty, as to continue their oppoſition againſt it, they are confident that a deſign ſo apparently beneficial to the Publick good, will not want the Encouragement and Protection of thoſe in whoſe Power it is to give it.

FINIS.

CLAREMONT.

Addreſs'd to the Right Honourable the

EARL of *CLARE.*

—Dryadum ſilvas, ſaltuſque ſequamur
Intactos, tua, Mæcenas, haud mollia juſſa. Virg.

LONDON:

Printed for *J. Tonſon*, at *Shakeſpear's-Head* over-against *Catherine-ſtreet* in the *Strand.* 1715.

THE

PREFACE.

THEY *that have seen those two excellent Poems of* Cooper's *Hill and* Windsor-Forrest; *the one by Sir* J. Denham, *the other by Mr.* Pope; *will show a great deal of Candour if they approve of this. It was writ upon giving the Name of* Claremont *to a* Villa, *now belonging to the Earl of* Clare. *The Situation is so agreeable and surprising, that it enclines one to think, some Place of this Nature put* Ovid *at first upon the Story of* Narcissus *and* Eccho. *'Tis probable he had observ'd some Spring rising amongst Woods and Rocks, where Ecchos were heard; and some Flower bending over the Stream and by Consequence reflected from it. After reading the Story in the Third Book of the* Metamorphosis, *'tis obvious to object (as an ingenious Friend has already done) that the renewing the Charms of a Nymph, of which* Ovid *had dispossess'd her,*

——vox tantum atque Ossa supersunt

is

is too great a Violation of Poetical Authority. I dare ſay the Gentleman who is meant wou'd have been well pleas'd to have found no Faults. There are not many Authors one can ſay the ſame of: Experience ſhows us every Day that there are Writers who cannot bear a Brother ſhou'd ſucceed, and the only Refuge from their Indignation is by being inconſiderable; upon which Reflection, this Thing ought to have a Pretence to their Favour.

They who wou'd be more inform'd of what relates to the Antient Britons, *and the* Druids *their Prieſts, may be directed by the Quotations to the Authors that have mention'd them.*

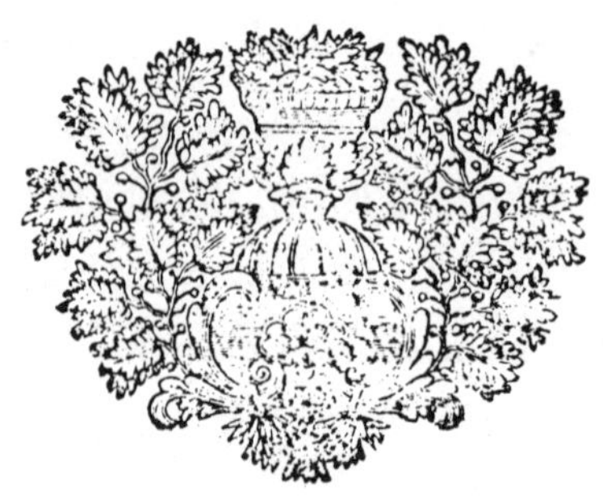

CLARE.

CLAREMONT.

Addreſs'd to the Right Honourable the

EARL of *CLARE.*

WHAT Frenzy has of late poſſeſs'd the Brain,
Tho' Few can write, yet Fewer can refrain!
So rank our Soyle, our Bards riſe in ſuch Store,
Their rich Retaining Patrons ſcarce are more.
The Laſt indulge the Fault, the Firſt commit;
And take off ſtill the Offall of their Wit.
So ſhameleſs, ſo abandon'd are their Ways;
They poche *Parnaſſus*, and lay Snares for Praiſe.

None ever can without Admirers live,
Who have a Penſion or a Place to give.
Great Miniſters ne'er fail of great Deſerts;
The Herald gives Them Blood; the Poet, Parts.
Senſe is of Courſe annex'd to Wealth and Pow'r;
No Muſe is proof againſt a golden Show'r.
Let but his Lordſhip write ſome poor Lampoon,
He's *Horac'd* up in Doggrel like his own.
Or if to rant in Tragick Rage he yields,
Falſe Fame crys----*Athens;* honeſt Truth----*Moorfields.*
Thus fool'd, he flounces on through Floods of Ink;
Flaggs with full Sail; and riſes but to ſink.

Some venal Pens ſo proſtitute the Bays,
Their Panegyricks laſh; their Satyrs praiſe.
So nauſeouſly, and ſo unlike they paint,
N—'s an *Adonis*; *M*—— *r* a Saint.
Metius with thoſe fam'd Heroes is compar'd
That led in Triumph *Porus* and *Tallard.*
But ſuch a ſhameleſs Muſe muſt Laughter move,
That aims to make *Salmoneus* vye with *Jove.*

To form great Works puts Fate it ſelf to Pain,
Ev'n Nature labours for a mighty Man.

And

And to perpetuate her Hero's Fame,
She ſtrains no leſs a Poet next to frame.
Rare as the Hero's, is the Poet's Rage;
Churchills and *Drydens* riſe but once an Age.
With Earthquakes tow'ring *Pindar*'s Birth begun;
And an Eclipſe produc'd * *Alcmena*'s Son:
The Sire of Gods o'er *Phœbus* caſt a Shade;
But, with a Hero, well the World repaid.

* Hercules.

No Bard for Bribes ſhou'd proſtitute his Vein;
Nor dare to Flatter where he ſhou'd Arraign.
To grant big *Thraſo* Valour, *Phormio*, Senſe,
Shou'd Indignation give, at leaſt Offence.

I hate ſuch Mercenaries, and wou'd try
From this Reproach to reſcue Poetry.
Apollo's Sons ſhou'd ſcorn the ſervile Art,
And to Court Preachers leave the fulſome Part.

What then—You'll ſay, Muſt no true Sterling paſs,
Becauſe impure Allays ſome Coin debaſe?
Yes, Praiſe, if juſtly offer'd, I'll allow;
And, when I meet with Merit, ſcribble too.

The Man who's honeſt, open, and a Friend,
Glad to oblige, uneaſie to offend:
Forgiving others, to himſelf ſevere;
Tho' earneſt, eaſie; civil, yet ſincere;
Who ſeldom but through great Good-nature errs;
Deteſting Fraud as much as Flatterers.
'Tis he my Muſe's Homage ſhou'd receive;
If I cou'd write, or *Holles* cou'd forgive.

But pardon, learned Youth, that I decline
A Name ſo lov'd by me, ſo lately Thine.
When *Pelham* you reſign'd, what cou'd repair
A Loſs ſo great, unleſs *Newcaſtle*'s Heir?
Hydaſpes that the *Aſian* Plains divides,
From his bright Urn in pureſt Chryſtal glides.
But when new gath'ring Streams enlarge his Courſe;
He's *Indus* nam'd, and rolls with mightier Force.
In fabl'd Floods of Gold his Current flows,
And Wealth on Nations, as he runs, beſtows.

Direct me, *Clare*, to name ſome nobler Muſe,
That for her Theme thy late *Receſs* may chuſe.
Such bright Deſcriptions ſhall the Subject dreſs;
Such vary'd Scenes, ſuch pleaſing Images;

That

That Swains ſhall leave their Lawns, and Nymphs their [Bow'rs,
And quit *Arcadia* for a Seat like yours.

But ſay, who ſhall attempt th' advent'rous Part
Where Nature borrows Dreſs from *Vanbrook*'s Art.
If, by *Apollo* taught, he touch the Lyre,
Stones mount in Columns, Palaces aſpire,
And Rocks are animated with his Fire.
'Tis he can Paint in Verſe thoſe riſing Hills,
Their gentle Vallies, and their ſilver Rills:
Cloſe Groves, and op'ning Glades with Verdure ſpread,
Flow'rs ſighing Sweets, and Shrubs that Balſam bleed.
With gay Variety the Proſpect crown'd,
And all the bright *Horiſon* ſmiling round.

Whilſt I attempt to tell how antient Fame
Records from whence the *Villa* took its Name.

In Times of old, when *Britiſh* Nymphs were known
To love no foreign Faſhions like their own;
When Dreſs was monſtrous, and Fig-leaves the Mode,
And Quality put on no Paint but * Woade.
Of *Spaniſh* Red unheard was then the Name;
For Cheeks were only taught to bluſh by Shame.

* *Glaſtum*. See *Pliny*. Ισάτις. See *Diaſcorides*.

No Beauty, to encreaſe her Crowd of Slaves,
Roſe out of Waſh, as *Venus* out of Waves.
Not yet Lead Comb was on the Toilett plac'd;
Not yet broad Eye-brows were reduc'd by Paſte:
No Shape-ſmith ſet up Shop, and drove a Trade
To mend the Work wiſe Providence had made.
Tyres were unheard of, and unknown the Loom,
And thrifty Silkworms ſpun for Times to come.
Bare Limbs were then the Marks of Modeſty;
All like *Diana* were below the Knee.

The Men appear'd a rough undaunted Race,
Surly in Show, unfaſhion'd in Addreſs.
* Upright in Actions, and in Thought ſincere;
And ſtrictly were the ſame they would appear.
Honour was plac'd in Probity alone;
For Villains had no Titles but their own.
None travell'd to return politely Mad;
But ſtill what Fancy wanted, Reaſon had.
Whatever Nature ask'd, their Hands cou'd give;
Unlearn'd in Feaſts, they only eat to live.
No Cook with Art encreas'd Phyſician's Fees;
Nor ſerv'd up Death in Soups and Friccacees.

* *Mores eis ſimplices, à verſutiâ & improbitate noſtræ tempeſtatis hominum longe remoti.* See Diod. Sic. Bib. Hiſt. L. IV. Verſ. Lat.

Their

Their Taſte was, like their Temper, unrefin'd;
For Looks were then the Language of the Mind.

E'er Right and Wrong, by turns, ſet Prices bore;
And Conſcience had its Rate like common Whore:
Or Tools to great Employments had Pretence;
Or Merit was made out by Impudence;
Or Coxcombs look'd aſſuming in Affairs;
And humble Friends grew haughty Miniſters.

In thoſe good Days of Innocence, here ſtood
Of Oaks, with Heads unſhorn, a ſolemn Wood,
Frequented by the * *Druids*, to beſtow
Religious Honours on the † Miſſelto.

The Naturaliſts are puzzel'd to explain
How Trees did firſt this Stranger entertain:
Whether the buſie Birds engraft it there;
Or elſe ſome Deity's myſterious Care,
As *Druids* thought; for when the blaſted Oak
By Lightning falls, this Plant eſcapes the Stroak.

* *Jam per ſe roborum eligunt lucos.* Plin. L. XVI.
† *Et nihil habent Druidæ viſco, & arbore in quâ gignatur, ſi modò ſit robur, ſacratius.* Plin. ibid.
Et Viſcum Druida. Ovid.

So

So when the *Gauls* the Tow'rs of *Rome* defac'd,
And Flames drove forward with outragious Waſte;
Jove's favour'd Capitol uninjur'd ſtood:
So Sacred was the Manſion of a God.

Shades honour'd by this Plant the *Druids* choſe,
Here, for the bleeding Victims, Altars roſe.
To * *Hermes* oft they paid their Sacrifice;
Parent of Arts, and Patron of the Wiſe.
Good Rules in mild Perſwaſions they convey'd;
Their Lives confirming what their Lectures ſaid.
None violated Truth, invaded Right;
Yet had few Laws, but Will and Appetite.
The People's Peace they ſtudy'd, and profeſt
No † Politicks but Publick Intereſt.
Hard was their Lodging, homely was their Food;
For all their Luxury was doing Good.

No Miter'd *Prieſt* did then with *Princes* vie,
Nor, o'er his Maſter, claim Supremacy;
Nor were the Rules of Faith allow'd more pure,
For being ſev'ral Centuries obſcure.

* *Deum maximè Mercurium colunt: Hunc omnium inventorem artium ferunt: Poſt hunc, Jovem, Apollinem &c.* Cæſ.

† *De republicâ, niſi per concilium, loqui non conceditur.* Cæſ. Lib. VI.

None loſt their Fortunes, forfeited their Blood,
For not believing what None underſtood.
Nor Symony, nor *Sine-Cure* were known;
Nor wou'd the Bee work Honey for the Drone.
Nor was the Way invented, to diſmiſs
Frail *Abigals* with fat *Pluralities*.

But then in Fillets bound, a hallow'd *Band*
Taught how to tend the Flocks, and till the Land:
Cou'd tell what Murrains in what Months begun,
And how the † Seaſons travell'd with the Sun:
When his dim Orb ſeem'd wading through the Air,
They told that Rain on dropping Wings drew near;
And that the Winds their bellowing Throats wou'd try,
When redd'ning Clouds reflect his Blood-ſhot Eye.

All their Remarks on Nature's Laws, require
More Lines than wou'd ev'n *Alpin*'s Readers tire.

This Sect in ſacred Veneration held
Opinions, by the *Samian Sage* reveal'd;
That Matter no Annihilation knows,
But wanders from Theſe Tenements to Thoſe.

† *Multa præterea de ſideribus, & eorum motu, de rerum natura &c.* Cæſ.

For when the *Plaſtick* Particles are gone,
They rally in ſome Species like their own.
The Self-ſame Atoms, if new jumbl'd, will
In Seas be reſtleſs, and in Earth be ſtill;
Can, in the Trufle, furniſh out a Feaſt;
And nauſeate, in the ſcaly Squill, the Taſte.
Thoſe falling Leaves that wither with the Year,
Will, in the next, on other Stems appear.
The Sap that now forſakes the burſting Bud,
In ſome new Shoot will circulate green Blood.
The Breath to Day that from the Jaſmin blows,
Will, when the Seaſon offers, ſcent the Roſe;
And thoſe bright Flames that in Carnations glow,
E'er long will blanch the Lilly with a Snow.

They hold that Matter muſt be ſtill the ſame;
And varies but in Figure and in Name.
And that the * Soul not dies, but ſhifts her Seat;
New Rounds of Life to run; or paſt, repeat.
Thus when the Brave and Virtuous ceaſe to live;
In Beings brave and virtuous they † revive.

* *Imprimis hoc volunt perſuadere, non interire animas, ſed ab aliis poſt mortem tranſire ad alios.* Cæſ.

† *Et vos Barbaricos ritus*——
Sacrorum Druidæ——
——*rediturae parcere vitæ.*
—— *regit idem ſpiritus artus:* Lucan. Lib. I.

Again

Again ſhall *Romulus* in *Naſſau* reign;
Great *Numa*, in a *Brunſwick* Prince, ordain
Good Laws; and *Halcyon* Years ſhall huſh the World [again.

The Truths of old Traditions were their Theme;
Or Gods deſcending in a Morning Dream.
Paſs'd Acts they cited; and to come, foretold;
And cou'd Events, not ripe for Fate, unfold.
Beneath the ſhady Covert of an Oak,
In † Rhymes uncooth, prophetick Truths they ſpoke.
Attend then *Clare*; nor is the Legend long;
The Story of thy *Villa* is their § Song.

The fair *Montano*, of the *Sylvan* Race,
Was with each Beauty bleſs'd, and ev'ry Grace.
His Sire, green *Faunus*, Guardian of the Wood;
His Mother, a ſwift *Naiad* of the Flood.
Her Silver Urn ſupply'd the neighb'ring Streams,
A darling Daughter of the bounteous *Thames*.

Not lovelier ſeem'd *Narciſſus* to the Eye;
Nor, when a Flower, cou'd boaſt more Fragrancy.

† *Et magnum numerum verſuum ediſcere dicuntur.* Cæſ.
§ *Superſtitione vanâ Druidæ canebant, &c.* Tacit. L. IV.

His

His Skin might with the Down of Swans compare,
More ſmooth than Pearl; than Mountain Snow more
In Shape ſo Poplars, or the Cedars pleaſe: [fair.
But Thoſe are not ſo ſtreight; nor graceful Theſe.
His flowing Hair in unforc'd Ringlets hung;
Tuneful his Voice, perſuaſive was his Tongue.
The haughtieſt Fair ſcarce heard without a Wound,
But ſunk to Softneſs at the melting Sound.

The fourth bright *Luſtre* had but juſt begun
To ſhade his bluſhing Cheeks with doubtful Down.
All Day he rang'd the Woods, and ſpread the Toils,
And knew no Pleaſures but in *Sylvan* Spoils.
In vain the Nymphs put on each pleaſing Grace;
Too cheap the Quarry ſeem'd, too ſhort the Chace.
For tho' Poſſeſſion be th' undoubted View;
To ſeize, is far leſs Pleaſure than purſue.
Thoſe Nymphs that yield too ſoon, their Charms impair,
And prove at laſt but deſpicably Fair.
His own Undoing Glutton *Love* decrees;
And palls the Appetite, he meant to pleaſe.
His ſlender Wants too largely he ſupplies:
Thrives on ſhort Meals, but by Indulgence dies.

A Grott there was with hoary Moſs o'ergrown,
Rough with rude Shells, and arch'd with mouldring Stone;
Sad Silence reigns within the loanſom Wall;
And weeping Rills but whiſper as they fall.
The claſping Ivys up the Ruin creep;
And there the Bat, and drowſie Beetle ſleep.

This Cell ſad *Eccho* choſe, by Love betray'd,
A fit Retirement for a mourning Maid.
Hither fatigu'd with Toil, the *Sylvan* flies
To ſhun the Calenture of ſultry Skies:
But feels a fiercer Flame, Love's keeneſt Dart
Finds through his Eyes a Paſſage to his Heart.
Penſive the *Virgin* ſate with folded Arms,
Her Tears but lending Luſter to her Charms.
With Pity he beholds her wounding Woes;
But wants himſelf the Pity he beſtows.

Oh whether of a Mortal born! he cries;
Or ſome fair Daughter of the diſtant Skies;
That, in Compaſſion leave your Chryſtal Sphere,
To guard ſome favour'd Charge, and wander here.
Slight not my Suit, nor too ungentle prove;
But pity One, a Novice yet in Love.

If Words avail not; ſee my ſuppliant Tears;
Nor diſregard thoſe dumb Petitioners.

From his Complaint the Tyrant Virgin flies,
Aſſerting all the Empire of her Eyes.

Full thrice three Days he lingers out in Grief,
Nor ſeeks from Sleep, or Suſtenance, Relief.
The Lamp of Life now caſts a glimm'ring Light;
The meeting Lids his ſetting Eyes benight.
What Force remains, the hapleſs Lover tries;
Invoking thus his kindred Deities.

Haſte, Parents of the Flood, your Race to mourn;
With Tears repleniſh each exhauſted Urn.
Retake the Life you gave, but let the Maid
Fall a juſt Victim to an injur'd Shade.
More he endeavour'd; but the Accents hung
Half form'd, and ſtopp'd unfiniſh'd on his Tongue.

For him the *Graces* their ſad Vigils keep;
Love broke his Bow, and wiſh'd for Eyes to weep.

What

What Gods can do, the mournful *Faunus* tries;
A Mount erecting where the *Sylvan* lies.
The Rural Pow'rs the wond'rous Pile ſurvey,
And piouſly their diff'rent Honours pay.
Th' Aſcent, with verdant Herbage *Pales* ſpread;
And Nymphs transform'd to Laurels, lent their Shade.
Her Stream a *Naiad* from the Baſis pours;
And *Flora* ſtrows the Summit with her Flowers.
Alone Mount *Latmos* claims Pre-eminence,
When Silver *Cynthia* lights the World from thence.

Sad *Eccho* now laments her Rigour, more
Than for *Narciſſus* her looſe Flame before.
Her Fleſh to Sinew ſhrinks, her Charms are fled;
All Day in rifted Rocks ſhe hides her Head.
Soon as the Ev'ning ſhows a Sky ſerene,
Abroad ſhe ſtrays, but never to be ſeen.
And ever as the weeping *Naiads* name
Her Cruelty, the Nymph repeats the ſame.
With them ſhe joins, her Lover to deplore,
And haunts the lonely Dales, he rang'd before.
Her Sex's Privilege ſhe yet retains;
And tho' to Nothing waſted, *Voice* remains.

So ſung the *Druids*----then with Rapture fir'd,
Thus utter what the * *Delphick* God inſpir'd.

E'er twice ten Centuries ſhall fleet away,
A *Brunſwick* Prince ſhall *Britain*'s Scepter ſway.
No more fair *Liberty* ſhall mourn her Chains;
The *Maid* is reſcu'd, her lov'd *Perſeus* reigns.
From † *Jove* he comes, the Captive to reſtore;
Nor can the Thunder of his *Sire* do more.
Religion ſhall dread nothing but Diſguiſe;
And Juſtice need no Bandage for her Eyes.
Britannia ſmiles, nor fears a foreign Lord;
Her Safety to ſecure, Two Powers accord,
Her *Neptune*'s Trident, and her *Monarch*'s Sword.
Like him, ſhall his *Auguſtus* ſhine in Arms,
Tho' Captive to his *Carolina*'s Charms.
Ages with future Heroes She ſhall bleſs;
And *Venus* once more found an *Alban* Race.

Then ſhall a *Clare* in Honour's Cauſe engage:
Example muſt reclaim a graceleſs Age.
Where Guides themſelves for Guilty Views miſ-lead;
And Laws ev'n by the Legiſlators bleed

* *Et partim auguriis, partim conjecturâ, quæ eſſent futura, &c.* Cic. de Divinatione.
† *Son of* Jupiter *and* Danae.

His

His brave Contempt of State ſhall teach the Proud,
None but the Virtuous are of Noble Blood.
For *Tyrants* are but *Princes* in Diſguiſe,
Tho' ſprung by long Deſcents from *Ptolomies*.
Right he ſhall Vindicate, good Laws defend;
The firmeſt Patriot, and the warmeſt Friend.
Great *Edward*'s * Order early He ſhall wear;
New Light reſtoring to the ſully'd *Star*.
Oft will his Leiſure this *Retirement* chuſe,
Still finding future Subjects for the Muſe,
And to record the *Sylvan*'s fatal Flame,
The *Place* ſhall live in Song; and *Claremont* be the Name.

* *Theologi & Vates erant apud eos, Druidas ipſi vocant, qui à victimarum extis de futuris divinant.* Diod. Sic. Lat. Ver.

FINIS.